RE Weller, Stella

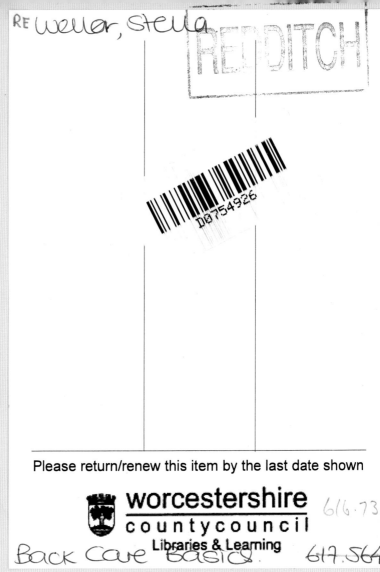
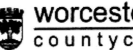

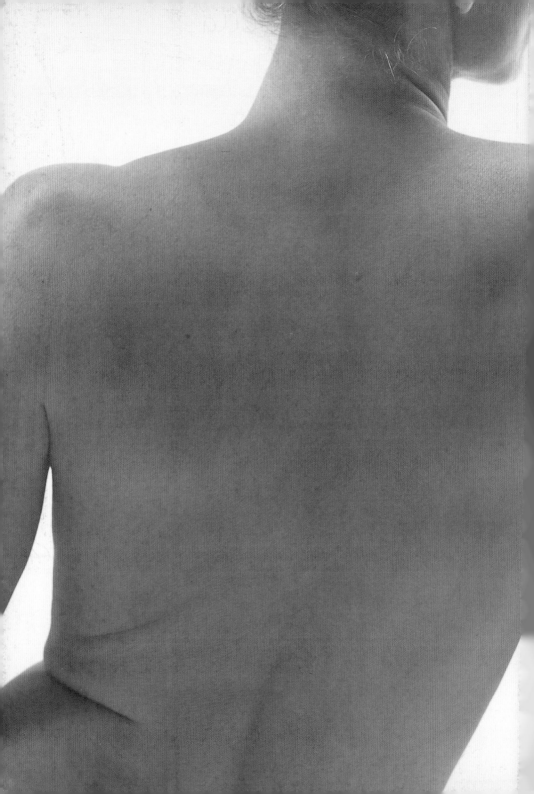

A Pyramid Health Paperback

Back care
basics

Stella Weller

hamlyn

To Fred and Pat with love.

An Hachette Livre UK Company
www.hachettelivre.co.uk

A Pyramid Paperback

First published in Great Britain in 2009 by
Hamlyn, a division of Octopus Publishing Group Ltd
2–4 Heron Quays, London E14 4JP
www.octopusbooks.co.uk

Distributed in the U.S. and Canada by Octopus Books USA:
c/o Hachette Book Group USA
237 Park Avenue
New York NY 10017

This material was previously published as *The Better Back Book*

ISBN 978-0-600-61811-9

A CIP catalogue record for this book is available from the
British Library

Printed and bound in China

10 9 8 7 6 5 4 3 2 1

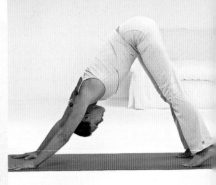

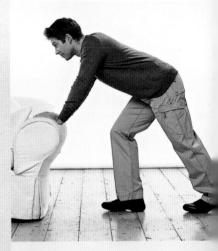

NOTE

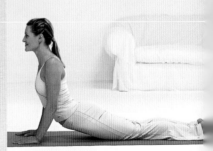

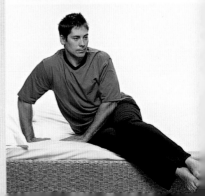

contents

introduction 6

understanding your spine 8

managing back pain 26

prevention is better than cure 44

exercises for a better back 58

back programmes 106

glossary 122

index 124

acknowledgements 128

introduction

Have you ever consulted a doctor about backache? Do you suffer from persistent back pain that lasts for at least 24 hours? Have you taken time off work because of a back problem?

If so, you are not alone. According to the World Health Organization, some form of back pain affects as many as 80 per cent of people at some time during their lives and results in significant costs for both individuals and society. In Britain, back pain is estimated to cost the country and business up to £6 billion in lost production every year and in the USA the figure is thought to be as high as $85 billion.

Dismaying though these statistics may be, help and hope are nevertheless at hand. This book shows you, through carefully chosen exercises, how you can improve your posture and strengthen your muscles both to prevent back problems developing and to treat existing back pain.

If you begin to practise better postural habits and also incorporate the simple exercises that are described in this book into your daily activities – starting with the beginners' exercises and working through them – you should notice improvements in as little as two weeks.By following the full 20-minute programme of exercises as outlined on pages 108–113 at least every other day, or doing a shortened version along with integrating some of the other exercises into your daily life, you will notice marked improvements in both how you feel and function within as little as four to six weeks from starting.

Reading through the different sections, you'll see that this book:

- explains the different types of back pain and how they are caused
- tells you how to prevent injury through adopting correct posture, appropriate exercise and lifestyle changes
- describes how to treat acute and chronic back pain safely, emphasizing self-help care wherever possible
- contains illustrated step-by-step exercises to strengthen the back and relieve discomfort. It includes exercises based on Pilates, yoga and the Alexander Technique
- provides a series of programmes for regular practice that can be incorporated into your daily routine.

No matter where you are, you have at your disposal some of the best 'tools' for helping you to acquire and maintain a strong and healthy back. They include your body, your mental resources – such as the ability to concentrate and to visualize – and also your breath (see pages 38–39).

The background information in this book, along with the exercises and techniques, will train you in the use of these resources. I encourage you to use them regularly and judiciously. This will enable you to be an informed, active participant in the best long-term plan for a problem-free back.

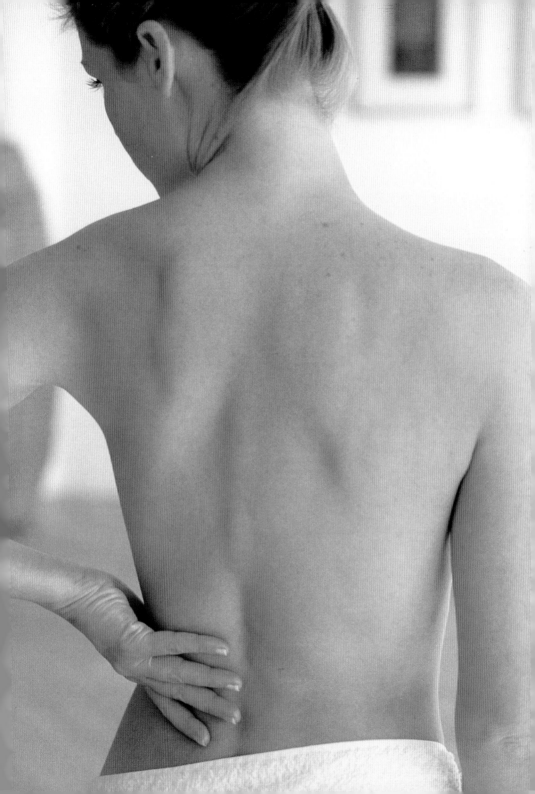

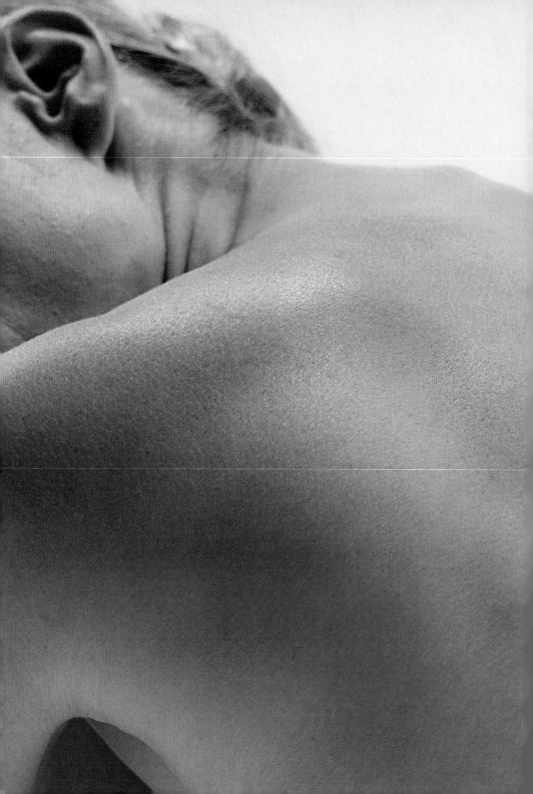

understanding
your spine

Your spine is a mechanical marvel. Although you do not need to be burdened with unnecessary technical details in order to know how best to take care of it, a basic understanding of its functions and structure is worth while. This will help you to better appreciate why certain postures, movements and actions are potentially injurious, while others promote a sense of wellbeing and help to prevent problems from arising. This chapter will also introduce you to the rationale behind the choice of exercises offered in this book. For all these reasons, please take a few minutes to read the following pages.

how the back works

The spine, also called the vertebral column or backbone, provides a strong, flexible support for the head and trunk. It also protects the spinal cord and serves as a point of attachment for the ribs, pelvis and muscles of the back.

Usually accounting for about two-fifths of the total height of the body, the spine is composed of 33 bones, called vertebrae, piled one upon another. These are named according to the position they occupy: there are 7 cervical (neck), 12 thoracic (chest), 5 lumbar (loin), 5 sacral (fused to form the sacrum) and usually 4 coccygeal (fused to form the coccyx, or tailbone) vertebrae. Between the sacrum and the hip bone (ilium) is the sacroiliac joint, which transmits the body's weight to the legs.

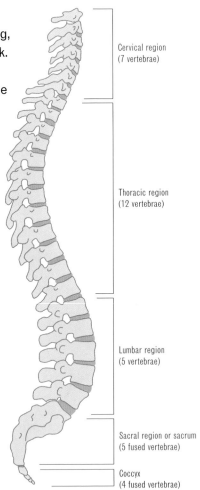

Cervical region
(7 vertebrae)

Thoracic region
(12 vertebrae)

Lumbar region
(5 vertebrae)

Sacral region or sacrum
(5 fused vertebrae)

Coccyx
(4 fused vertebrae)

The spine is made up of 33 vertebrae stacked on top of each other. Running through its centre, protected by the surrounding bone, is the spinal cord – the primary route for signals between the body and the brain.

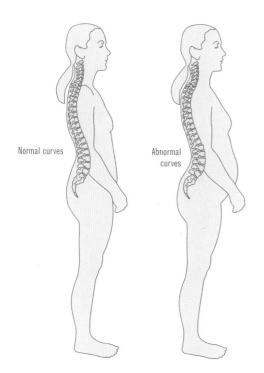

Normal curves

Abnormal curves

normal curves

If you look at the spine from the side, you will see that it consists of four curves. The cervical and lumbar areas curve forwards (are convex anteriorly), while the thoracic and sacral areas curve backwards (are concave anteriorly). These gentle curves are important because they increase the strength of the backbone, help to maintain balance in the upright position, absorb shock during walking and help to protect the spine from injury when jumping or falling.

The normal spine curves naturally in an S-shape – in at the neck, out at the shoulders, in again at waist level and outwards at the base. This shape makes the spine flexible and able to withstand the stresses and strains of everyday life.

nerves and spinal cord

Running through the central canal formed by the stacked vertebrae from the base of the brain to the first lumbar vertebra is the spinal cord. This cylinder of nerve tissue is an extension of the brain and acts as the main route for sensory information passing between the brain and the body. Along the length of the spinal cord, 31 pairs of nerves branch out through openings between the vertebrae called foramina. These nerves carry commands from the brain to organs and muscles, as well as messages about temperature, touch and pain back to the spinal cord and brain.

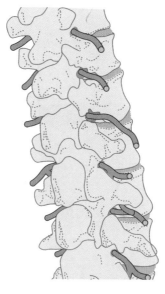

Thirty-one pairs of nerves branch out from the spinal cord. They emerge from either side through gaps between adjacent vertebrae.

a typical vertebra

Although vertebrae in different regions up and down the spine vary in size, shape and detail, they typically consist of two essential parts: a solid cylindrical segment known as the vertebral body at the front, and a knobbly, roughly triangular segment known as the vertebral arch (or neural arch) at the back. The body, which has flat upper and lower surfaces, known as end plates, is convex in front and flattened at the back. The flattened area forms the front of the spinal canal through which the spinal cord and nerve roots pass. The arch surrounds the rest of the spinal canal and gives protection to the structures within it. It also has two upper and lower surfaces called facets. The lower facets of one vertebra glide along those of the vertebra below, limiting the motion of one relative to its neighbour and preventing one from slipping off the other. Facets connect the rear portions of vertebrae to form joints.

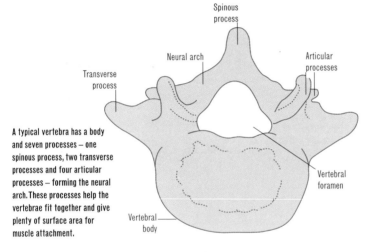

Spinous process

Neural arch

Articular processes

Transverse process

Vertebral foramen

Vertebral body

A typical vertebra has a body and seven processes – one spinous process, two transverse processes and four articular processes – forming the neural arch. These processes help the vertebrae fit together and give plenty of surface area for muscle attachment.

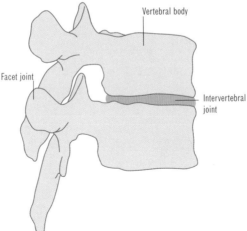

Vertebral body

Facet joint

Intervertebral joint

There are three joints between each pair of neighbouring lumbar vertebrae – the intervertebral joint between adjacent bodies and two facet joints between the processes. The facet joints hold the intervertebral joint in place and stop it being twisted too much or shifted forwards.

intervertebral discs

From the second cervical vertebra right down to the sacrum, the bodies of adjacent vertebrae are separated by intervertebral discs. Each disc has a tough outer fibrous ring and an inner, soft, very elastic core. The discs cushion the vertebrae and permit movements of the spine while absorbing vertical shock. The inner, jelly-like core of the disc can readily absorb fluid and swell. Although this is normally counteracted by the weight of the body pressing the discs between the vertebrae, at night while we are asleep the swelling process meets no resistance and the discs expand. This explains why we are somewhat taller when we get up in the morning than we are towards the end of the day.

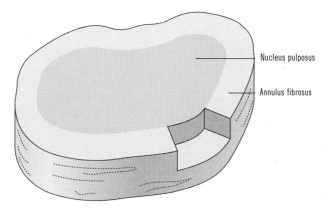

A normal intervertebral disc has a tough, elastic shell (annulus fibrosus) that protects the soft, jelly-like interior (nucleus pulposus). The upper and lower surfaces have a cartilaginous layer known as the end plate.

Nucleus pulposus

Annulus fibrosus

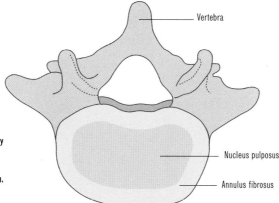

Discs cushion vertebrae. They are firmly attached to those above and below and can withstand much compression. They do not actually slip but they can bulge or rupture.

Vertebra

Nucleus pulposus

Annulus fibrosus

spinal reinforcements

Vertebrae are joined to one another by ligaments – these are tough bands of fibrous tissue, which closely surround the bodies and connect the arches. The ligaments keep the vertebrae in alignment and help to prevent damage from excessive movements. Flexible fibrous cords called tendons attach the muscles of the back to the spine.

Furthermore, the spine is stabilized by powerful muscles attached to the vertebrae, the pelvis and the back of the chest wall. These work together to keep the spine well aligned yet mobile. During exertion, the muscles contract and cause a stiffening of the spine, enabling it to tolerate the added stress caused.

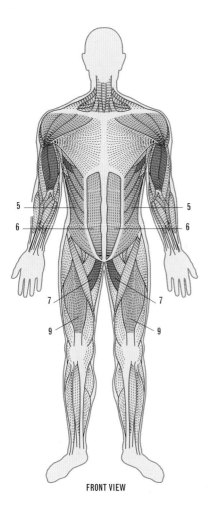

FRONT VIEW

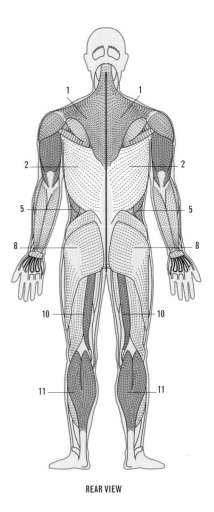

REAR VIEW

THE SPINAL SUPPORT MUSCLES

1 Trapezius – runs down the back of the neck and along the shoulders. It is used to extend the head.

2 Latissimus dorsi – runs from the lower chest to the lumbar region. It draws the arm backwards, pulls the shoulder down and back and the body upwards.

3 Erector spinae (not shown) – this important muscle is at the back of the neck, chest and abdomen. It extends the spine and holds the body upright. When it acts on one side only it bends the spine to that side.

4 Transversus abdominis (not shown) – a deep internal muscle that runs across the abdomen. It holds the internal organs in place.

5 External oblique – side muscle of the abdomen. It compresses the abdomen and is used when moving the torso in any direction.

6 Rectus abdominis – runs vertically down the front of the abdomen, supporting the internal organs and drawing the front of the pelvis upwards.

7 Adductor – this inner thigh muscle draws the leg inwards.

8 Gluteus maximus – forms the buttocks. It is important for maintaining an upright posture and in walking, running and jumping.

9 Quadriceps – runs down the middle of the front of the thigh. It acts in opposition to the semitendinosus.

10 Semitendinosus – also known as the hamstrings. It runs down the middle of the back of the thigh and is used to extend the thigh and flex the knee.

11 Gastrocnemius – forming the greater part of the calf, this muscle runs down the back of the lower leg and is used in walking and running.

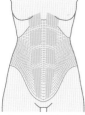
Transversus abdominis

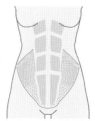
Internal obliques

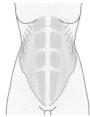
External obliques

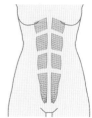
Rectus abdominis

the abdominal muscles

Indirect spinal reinforcement is also provided by four sets of abdominal muscles (see above). The abdominals surround the lower torso and connect the pelvis to the ribs, stabilizing the spine and allowing the body to bend and twist. The outermost layer, the rectus abdominis, is the easiest to activate but it needs to be controlled by the deeper layers.

other related structures

In addition to the many ligaments, tendons and muscles mentioned here, the spine receives indirect support from the leg muscles, notably the quadriceps at the front of the thighs and the hamstrings (also known as the semitendinosus) at the back of the thighs. These muscles influence the degree of pelvic tilt and so have a bearing on your posture.

pelvic ring

The spine is balanced on an undulating base that is known as the pelvic ring or pelvic girdle. This is the body's chief weight-transmitting structure, connecting the upper body to the legs. It consists of the sacrum at the back and two innominate (hip) bones, which are connected to the femurs (thigh bones). Together, these bones form five joints: two sacroiliac joints at the base of the spine; two hip joints where the hip bones connect with the legs, and the symphysis pubis where the two hip bones join in front.

During normal standing or sitting, the ligaments of the sacroiliac joints and the pelvic ring are somewhat loose. When weight-bearing occurs, however, the pressure extended down through the spinal column causes the sacroiliac ligaments to tighten, changing the pelvic ring from a loose, or neutral, structure to one that makes for greater stability.

A second key characteristic of the pelvic ring is that its degree of tilt affects the curvature of the spinal column above. Any change

in the angle of the sacral portion of the pelvis will thus determine posture. If the pelvic ring is in a balanced position, the spinal curves will be proportionately balanced and the posture safe. If, however, the pelvic ring is abnormally tilted, poor posture will result and the spine will consequently be more vulnerable to injury and pain.

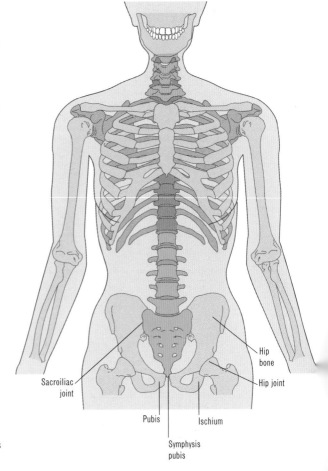

The basin-shaped pelvis at the base of the spine supports the upper half of the body and protects the abdominal organs. The tilt of the pelvis affects the curvature of the spine and thus influences posture.

Sacroiliac joint

Hip bone

Hip joint

Pubis

Ischium

Symphysis pubis

pelvic floor muscles

The pelvic floor is a group of muscles and ligaments situated at the bottom of the pelvis and forms a sling-like support for pelvic organs. Part of the floor (the perineum) may be seen externally as the area that lies between the thighs, from the anus to the external genitals.

Backache may sometimes be related to a weak or slack pelvic floor and the resulting effect on some of the internal structures, albeit indirectly.

One way to strengthen your pelvic floor muscles is to practise the Perineal Exercise (below) several times a day.

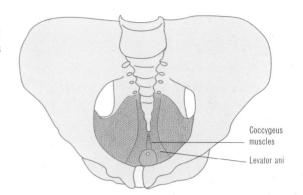

Coccygeus muscles

Levator ani

The pelvic floor muscles form a sling-like structure that supports the internal organs. A weak pelvic floor can lead to back pain and incontinence so it is important to exercise it.

perineal exercise

Strengthens the pelvic floor to provide an efficient support for structures within the torso
Enhances diaphragmatic breathing

1 Sit, lie or stand comfortably. Relax your jaw and breathe regularly through your nose.

2 Exhale and tighten your perineum (exterior region between the anus and the external genitals). Hold the tightness as long as your exhalation lasts. (Do not tighten your jaw.)

3 Inhale and relax. Breathe regularly and rest.

Repeat the exercise several times during the day.

VARIATION

Combine with visualization: imagine you are in a lift, going up to the tenth floor. As you exhale, start to tighten your perineum a little at a time and with control, to correspond with your trip to the tenth floor. Do not lose any muscle tension as you progress; let it accumulate. When your exhalation is complete, inhale and relax your perineum in stages, as you descend to the ground floor. Breathe regularly and rest. Choose the number of floors to match the length of your respirations.

BEGINNER
2 times; hold
3 to 4 seconds

INTERMEDIATE
3 times; hold
5 or more seconds

ADVANCED
4 times; hold
8 or more seconds

causes of pain

Although marvellous in its construction, and being both strong and flexible, the spine is nevertheless vulnerable to a myriad of disorders. Some conditions are simply due to the processes of wear and tear, while others are the effects of conditions such as infection, tumours, injuries, poor postural habits and even pregnancy. This section examines some of the more common causes of backache and back pain.

disc problems

The intervertebral discs (see page 13) can be traced as a source of some of the most familiar of all back ailments. The 'slipped disc' is, in fact, a disc from which the jelly-like contents are bulging or have even escaped their normal boundaries (herniated or prolapsed), causing the disc to impinge on neighbouring ligaments or nerves. Inflammation and pain may ensue from the pressure on these structures.

Although herniated (prolapsed) discs do not always cause problems, they can produce some bothersome symptoms that include numbness or tingling in the legs and also pain. Herniated discs are the most common cause of sciatica, which produces severe pain in the leg, along the course of the sciatic nerve, felt at the back of the thigh and along the inside of the leg.

Herniated discs are often the result of bad posture and poor body mechanics during daily activities, such as bending and lifting. They also occur as a consequence of injuries during sports, particularly those that involve running, jumping and twisting, or those requiring extreme flexibility, such as gymnastics. They can also occur because of degenerative changes as we grow older. With age, discs gradually lose water and become smaller, less springy and less effective as shock absorbers.

Herniated discs are usually diagnosed with the help of techniques such as MRI (magnetic resonance imaging). As a rule, recommended treatments are non-invasive and include rest, the judicious use of pain relievers, learning proper bending and lifting techniques, and general back care to reduce mechanical wear and tear. Surgery is usually reserved for cases in which other previous treatments have failed.

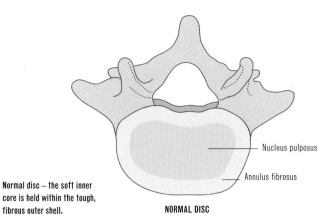

Normal disc – the soft inner
core is held within the tough,
fibrous outer shell.

NORMAL DISC

Nucleus pulposus

Annulus fibrosus

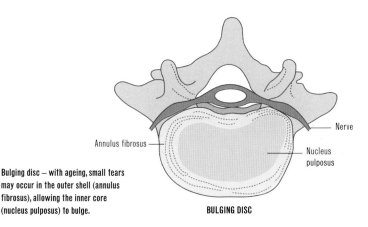

Bulging disc – with ageing, small tears
may occur in the outer shell (annulus
fibrosus), allowing the inner core
(nucleus pulposus) to bulge.

BULGING DISC

Annulus fibrosus

Nerve

Nucleus
pulposus

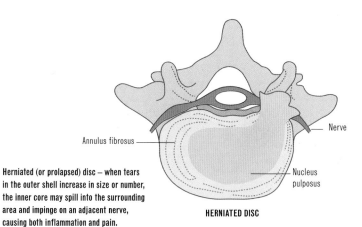

Herniated (or prolapsed) disc – when tears
in the outer shell increase in size or number,
the inner core may spill into the surrounding
area and impinge on an adjacent nerve,
causing both inflammation and pain.

HERNIATED DISC

Annulus fibrosus

Nerve

Nucleus
pulposus

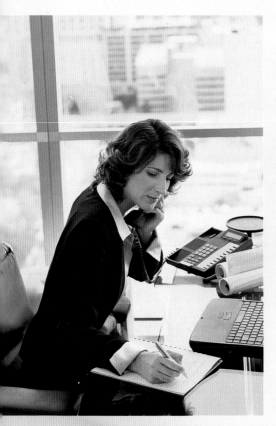

Take frequent breaks from repetitive work or prolonged awkward postures to do appropriate tension-relieving exercises.

also others such as the facet joints (see page 12); and rheumatoid arthritis, which can sometimes produce crippling deformities. Osteoarthritis-related degenerative changes in the spinal bones and joints, which are common among people over forty, are known as spondylosis. (The prefix 'spondyl' means vertebra.) They can result in an abnormal curvature of the thoracic (chest) spine in older people – a condition known as kyphosis.

For accurate diagnosis, X-rays are required. Treatments include: rest, immobilization, pain-relieving and anti-inflammatory medication, followed by graduated exercise and postural training by a physiotherapist. Surgery is necessary only in very extreme cases.

arthritis

The term arthritis refers to inflammation of a joint anywhere in the body, including the spine. The condition may result from, or be associated with, various disorders including infection, degenerative disease, metabolic disturbances and tumours.

Types of arthritis include: ankylosing (rheumatoid) spondylitis, a chronic progressive disease that usually affects the spine and adjacent structures; osteoarthritis, affecting mostly the weight-bearing joints, but

injury

Back pain of varying intensity and duration may arise from injury either to the bone itself, as occurs in fractures, or to muscles, tendons, ligaments or nerves.

Muscle tears may result from direct trauma or from overuse, as when participating in sports, or from prolonged awkward postures and poor body mechanics. When a muscle is strained ('pulled muscle') or torn, its blood vessels are also damaged and surrounding tissues become inflamed.

Muscle strains and tears often produce spasm – a sudden, intense, involuntary muscle contraction. Although such spasms can be painful, it is the body's natural mechanism for protecting injured tissue by temporarily splinting the part to limit movement for healing purposes.

Like muscles, ligaments supporting the joints of the back are also subject to injury. They can be overstretched or torn, from a fall for example, or from overuse as in activities such as ballet dancing or gymnastics. The spine's fibrous ligaments can also be damaged from the cumulative stress of habitual bad posture and poor body mechanics.

The type of damage known as a sprain often affects the ligaments that bind together the spine's facet joints (see page 12). This most often occurs in the lumbar area, although the sacroiliac joints (see page 16) are also vulnerable, particularly during a fall or a twisting action.

Precautions to take to prevent such injury include proper warming-up and stretching exercises before engaging in sports or other strenuous activities, and training and practice in correct lifting techniques, where applicable. Cumulative stress can be averted by attention to good postural habits and by taking frequent breaks from repetitive work to do appropriate tension-relieving exercises.

other causes of back pain

Back pain may result from changes in the bone itself, infections and tumours, and even from a natural process such as pregnancy. There are also certain specific conditions that may be diagnosed.

spondylolisthesis

In this condition one vertebra slips forward (subluxates) on top of another. This movement narrows the spinal canal through which the spinal cord passes, and encroaches on spinal nerves. Although it can occur anywhere along the spine, it most frequently involves the slipping of the bottom lumbar vertebra over the sacrum.

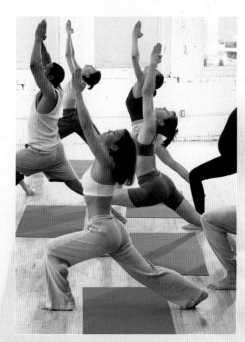

A normal part of any exercise class is the warming-up session at the beginning. Stretching may be done before or after the main activity to avoid injury.

Spondylolisthesis may be the result of trauma, a spinal fracture or arthritis. Its symptoms include mild low back pain, muscle spasm and sciatica, or it may produce no symptoms at all. Practising good postural habits and strengthening the muscles of the trunk are good preventive measures to take.

spondylolysis

Another condition with a similar name is spondylolysis. In this disorder, there is a separation or break of vertebral bone. It can occur because of an injury or as a result of long-term stress on the bone.

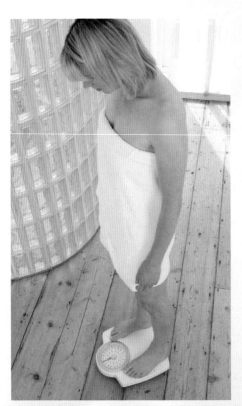

osteoporosis

Characterized by increased bone porosity, osteoporosis results from the bone breaking down faster than it is being formed. Most often this condition is found in women around the menopause; but osteoporosis is not uncommon among men with sedentary lifestyles. Bones become more brittle and fragile and therefore more vulnerable to fracture. Particularly problematic is bone loss in the spine where vertebrae can become compressed and fractures can occur. Deformities such as kyphosis (hunchback) may appear.

scoliosis

This sideways curvature of the spine may be present at birth or develop later in life. Most often it's seen in teenage girls, it can also result from habitual poor posture during growth and development.

tumours and infection

Back pain and related symptoms may arise from a wide range of diseases. These include tumours (both benign and malignant), disorders of the bladder, prostate gland, kidneys, large intestine, female reproductive organs, endocrine glands, such as the thyroid, and infections of bone and muscle.

Weight can be a factor in causing back pain. Being overweight can create extra pressure on the discs in the lumbar spine.

In pregnancy, the body becomes more flexible and it is especially important to guard against injury and take care not to overstrain the joints and muscles of the back.

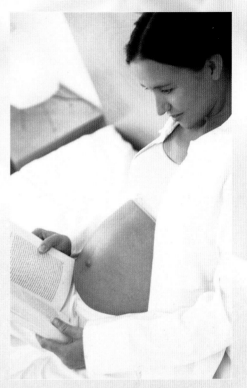

pregnancy

During pregnancy, the joints and ligaments become more relaxed than usual because of the action of a hormone called relaxin. This alters the mechanics of the sacroiliac and other joints, and increases the chances of injury such as strain or sprain or undue pressure on intervertebral discs. In addition, the extra abdominal weight increases the spine's lumbar arch as the buttocks push out to compensate. This understandably alters the body's centre of gravity and stresses lower back muscles.

inactivity

Prolonged sitting exerts greater than normal pressure on discs and puts the back at risk. Office workers, for example, whose work confines them to a desk or computer for many hours a day without periodic breaks, are vulnerable to back problems. So are people who are confined to bed through illness.

If the muscles of the back and abdomen are not exercised on a regular basis or the spine put through its range of motion, the back becomes especially vulnerable to various stresses. As a result, joints stiffen, ligaments and muscles overcontract, blood flow is restricted and any degeneration of vertebral joints is accelerated.

weight

Being over- or underweight is a risk factor for back pain. As already noted, the extra weight of pregnancy increases pressure on discs of the lumbar spine. On the other hand, extreme weight loss, as seen in conditions such as anorexia nervosa, may result in unusual pressure on nerves because of the loss of protective muscle tissue as well as lower bone density.

stress

In the 1970s, Dr Frederick Leboyer remarked that the state of our mind is a reflection of the state of our back. This observation is not as far-fetched

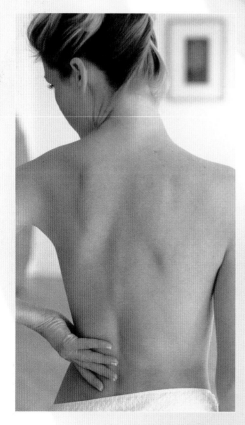

The lower back is a common site of chronic pain. Compression of lumbar vertebrae is a frequent cause, often due to poor posture and weak muscles.

chronic back pain

The most common cause of chronic back pain is compression of the lumbar vertebrae. When this occurs, the intervertebral discs shrink, the facet joints are jammed together and inflammation ensues, causing pain.

Compression of vertebrae may be the result of muscular imbalances. It may also be a consequence of weak muscles, especially those of the abdomen, which play a valuable supportive role. Or, it may occur because of habitual bad posture.

Prolonged sitting can cause disc compression, as can wearing shoes with high heels, which places unnatural stress on the spinal muscles and ligaments.

The ageing process can take its toll on the spinal structures: with age, intervertebral discs lose some of their moisture content and their outer rings become more brittle and so vulnerable to cracks. Fluid can then escape and place pressure on surrounding structures, such as nerves. Pain will follow.

who is at risk?

No one is immune to back pain. Even the fittest person among us may, at one time or another, be

as it may at first appear. Indeed, there are many documented cases to support it.

The experience of pain is influenced not only by physical factors, such as pressure on nerves, but also by religious beliefs, ethnicity and personality. Also playing a part in how we respond to pain stimuli are memory, attention, depression, fear and various causes of stress, such as job dissatisfaction. All of these factors increase tension in the body and so intensify and prolong back pain.

vulnerable to an occurrence that may put our back at risk. For some of us, even a sudden sneeze or forceful cough could result in back strain.

Certain occupations, however, pose greater risks than others. There are several categories of jobs that can seriously stress the back, such as those involving heavy lifting and twisting (for example, construction work, landscaping, nursing, fire fighting, commercial fishing and logging) and those requiring unrelieved prolonged sitting or standing (such as long-distance lorry and bus drivers, assembly-line workers, computer workers, librarians and accountants). Other employees at risk include postal workers, who spend long periods on their feet and may have to make sudden moves. And even those who do nothing at all but sit or lie on a couch for long periods watching television are at risk from their inactive lifestyles.

There are, of course, other causes of back pain and related problems. These include extra weight gained during pregnancy, trauma from a sports injury, car accident or fall, cumulative stress from years of poor postural habits, a congenital spinal defect or a disorder of mental origin, such as anxiety or depression.

SYMPTOMS QUESTIONNAIRE

The following questionnaire has been prepared to assist you in identifying factors that may be contributing to your back problem. You may find it's useful in building up an overall picture of how these factors can have a long-term impact on your functioning and wellbeing, and so the questionnaire could well motivate you to make constructive lifestyle changes. It may also better equip you for a visit to the doctor by providing ready answers for the questions that you may be asked.

• When did your current pain start?
• What do you think triggered the pain?

• What symptoms are you experiencing? Pain? Stiffness? Weakness? Numbness?
• Is the pain constant? Intermittent? Dull? Sharp? Shooting?
• Where is it located? Small of the back? Sacrum? Neck? Legs? Does it radiate to other parts of the body?
• Are your symptoms also generating other difficulties, such as bladder and bowel problems?
• What makes the pain worse or better? (Changing position? Sitting? Standing? Lying down? During sexual intercourse? When you're exposed to cold?)

• How do the symptoms interfere with your daily activities? (Specify activities.)
• Do your symptoms prevent you from having adequate sleep at night?
• Are your symptoms making you feel depressed? How?
• Have your symptoms abated, or worsened, since they first appeared (less frequent, less intense, or more so)?
• Have you been diagnosed with a health disorder, such as a thyroid or prostate gland problem, arthritis or osteoporosis?

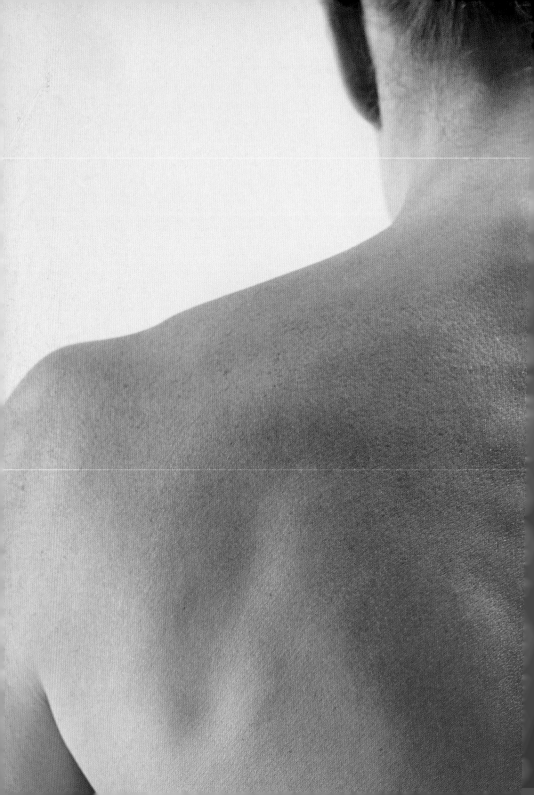

managing
back pain

Pain is a warning signal that helps to
protect the body from tissue damage. It is also
an experience and not merely a symptom. Pain is
whatever and wherever the sufferer says it is. In this
chapter you will gain some understanding of the pain
mechanism and find ways to deal with it, including
medical/surgical, complementary, self-help
and emergency measures.

pain control

Why is it that some people tolerate pain better than others? Although it is a universal experience, the degree to which you feel pain and how you react to it depends on many factors, such as previous encounters with pain or illness, as well as your own psychological, biological and cultural make-up.

the 'gate control' theory

The now classic spinal 'gate control' theory, which was first proposed in the 1960s by the Canadian psychologist Ronald Melzack and the British physiologist Patrick Wall, is a plausible and respected explanation. It suggests that there is a nervous system mechanism that, in effect, opens or closes a 'gate', controlling pain stimuli travelling to the brain where they are interpreted. This gate mechanism can be affected by certain psychological processes. For example, your attitude to the occurrence of pain can determine whether or not you will feel the pain and also to what extent. In addition, if you are stressed or anxious, your perception of the pain will tend to intensify.

This mechanism can be seen in action when a woman approaching childbirth uses breathing techniques in order to help relieve the stress and pain of labour. It can also be seen in athletes who are able to shut out the pain experienced during the physical exertion of a game or track event.

There are various ways of closing the spinal gate to block some of the painful stimuli from reaching the brain. These include conventional medication, surgery, physical therapy and electrical therapy, as well as complementary approaches.

physical therapy

The three commonly used physical techniques for the relief of back pain include traction, massage and direct applications of heat and/or cold.

Traction uses mechanical apparatus to stretch the back muscles and ligaments in order to relieve the pressure on spinal nerves and intervertebral discs.

Massage, and **heat and cold** are forms of cutaneous (skin) stimulation that draw their rationale from the gate control theory of pain transmission (see above). They work on the principle of blocking the passage of pain sensations to the brain and also on stimulating the production of endorphins, the chemicals that are the body's natural pain relievers.

All of these techniques generate nerve impulses that enter the spinal cord and brain with pain-relieving consequences.

psychological control of pain

The gate control theory proposes that psychological activities such as attention and suggestion can influence pain perception. We now know that psychological methods of pain control can decrease some kinds of pain from unbearable to more tolerable levels. Psychologists, psychiatrists and other specialists therefore are now using methods that involve suggestion, distraction, relaxation, biofeedback and similar techniques to help relieve pain. Some methods are described over the following pages.

complementary approaches

In addition to acupuncture, acupressure, chiropractic and osteopathy (see page 35), the disciplines considered particularly beneficial in bringing relief to people experiencing back problems include reflexology, Rolfing as well as the Feldenkrais Method.

Reflexology is based on the idea that there are reflex areas, or zones, on the hands and feet that are linked, through the nerves, to all the glands, organs and other vital structures of the body. Manipulating these areas with the thumb, finger or hand, using special techniques, is believed to relieve pain elsewhere in the body and promote relaxation and healing.

Rolfing is a system of body education and soft tissue manipulation that is designed to bring the body into good alignment. In order to restructure the body, a Rolfing practitioner presses firmly on various points using fingers, knuckles or elbows to help restore joint function, ease pain and speed up healing.

The **Feldenkrais Method** is a system of physical re-education that was designed to encourage body awareness, improve flexibility and enhance wellbeing. Feldenkrais practitioners believe that certain habitual postures and movements disrupt the healthy functioning of the nervous system. They teach students to identify these and avoid them. Gentle manipulation is also sometimes used in the Feldenkrais Method.

Practitioners of these three methods usually belong to a professional organization. To find a qualified practitioner in your area, look up pertinent organizations on the Internet; always ensure a practitioner is registered with a recognized professional body.

self-help care

In addition to the preventive strategies described in the next chapter, there are various approaches that you can use to treat back pain at home.

Experts agree that prevention and self-care bring better and more long-term results than any other approach to treatment for back pain. In many cases, given appropriate guidance and advice, you can look after your back at home without resorting to complex, costly equipment and procedures.

treating pain

The various methods currently used to relieve pain are generally based on the concept that signals of injury can be modified or even blocked at the earliest stages of transmission within the nervous system. Their aim is to stimulate endorphin production, alter the perception of pain and raise pain tolerance.

medicines

Some of the remedies that are most frequently taken to relieve back pain belong to a group of medicines known as NSAIDs (pronounced 'en-sayds'). These non-steroidal anti-inflammatory drugs include the widely used medicines aspirin and ibuprofen, both of which are available over the counter without a doctor's prescription. NSAIDs have a dual action: they reduce inflammation and relieve pain.

Also widely available over the counter is paracetamol. This is a simple analgesic (pain reliever) that does not in itself reduce the inflammation that contributes to the pain.

Another group of medicines used to alleviate back pain are the skeletal muscle relaxants. An example is cyclobenzaprine (also known by its brand name – Flexeril), which is sometimes prescribed for pain resulting from muscle spasms associated with injury. It is usually used in conjunction with rest, physical therapy and complementary relief measures such as breathing and relaxation exercises: Progressive Relaxation (see pages 76–77), A Healing Visualization (see page 37) and the Anti-anxiety Breath (see page 39) are three examples of these exercises.

People who are in pain, especially if it is constant or long term, are prone to depression. Antidepressant agents are therefore sometimes prescribed as

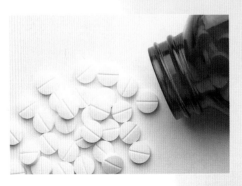

NSAIDs, which reduce inflammation and relieve pain, are available over the counter without a prescription.

an adjunct to other pain-relieving medication.

For severe back problems, where simpler forms of treatment have not worked, an injection may be given. Sometimes doctors administer a corticosteroid that is mixed with a local anaesthetic. The corticosteroid reduces inflammation by limiting the body's production of prostaglandins (active biological substances that affect many tissues and organs). The anaesthetic temporarily 'deadens' or 'freezes' the tissues to ease the pain of both the injection and the complaint itself.

All medicines can produce unwanted side-effects, including skin rash, stomach upsets, headache, drowsiness, dizziness, fatigue and insomnia. Some can be addictive. Others should be avoided by people with certain medical conditions. Consult your doctor or pharmacist before taking any medications.

CAUTION
- **Do not take aspirin and ibuprofen together. They may work against one another and also increase the likelihood of side-effects.**

surgery

No more than 5 per cent of all back pain sufferers are likely to benefit from surgery. In general, surgical procedures are reserved for cases that have not responded successfully to other, non-invasive, treatments. It may be vital, however, for those whose back pain is caused by a serious condition such as cancer or a fractured vertebra.

Surgical procedures include **laminectomy**, in which pieces (laminae) of vertebrae are removed, **discectomy**, in which portions of a disc are removed, and **spinal fusion**, in which two or more vertebrae are joined together permanently.

If surgery has been recommended for your back problem, do learn as much as you can about the procedure from your doctor or other reliable professional source. If in doubt, ask for a second opinion before going ahead.

cold and heat

Ice

For the first day or two after the appearance of minor back pain, ice may be applied to the affected area both to induce numbness and to reduce any swelling. One good way to do this is to put crushed ice and a little water in a plastic bag, seal it well, cover it with a towel and apply it to the affected area. A bag of frozen peas or sweetcorn kernels also works well for this, as do refrigerated towels.

To avoid damage to the skin and underlying tissues, apply the ice for not more than 15 to 20 minutes at a time, allowing 20 to 40 minutes between applications.

Three or four applications a day should be enough to offer relief.

CAUTIONS

- Do not use cold applications if you are very sensitive to cold or if you have Raynaud's phenomenon (a disorder of the blood vessels in the fingers and toes that causes them to contract suddenly in response to cold or emotional stress).
- Be cautious also in using this treatment if you have rheumatoid arthritis.
- Try not to doze off while an ice pack is in place.

Heat

After using ice for about a 48-hour period, you may try an application of moist heat to relax tense muscles and ease stiffness. Apply heat for 20 minutes about twice a day using warm, moist towels or take a warm shower or bath.

CAUTIONS

- Do not use heat if your back pain was caused by a blow to the back or by a fall or other accident.

Massage contributes to pain relief by reducing muscle tension and promoting relaxation.

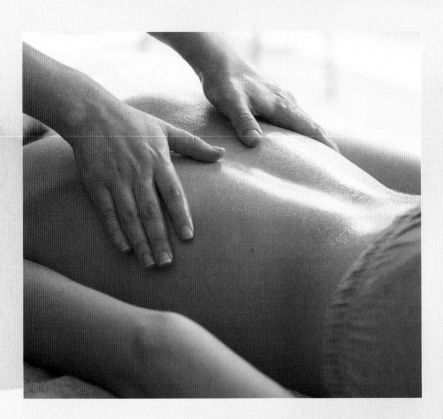

massage

By increasing blood flow to the affected area, massage facilitates the elimination of noxious wastes. It also reduces muscle tension and aids relaxation, and so contributes to pain relief.

Of all the available massage methods, the human touch is perhaps the most therapeutic of all. But various massage machines can also be effective. They vary from vibrating cushions to hand-held devices. They give only superficial massage but are nevertheless useful in reducing muscle tension and spasm, and promoting relaxation.

CAUTIONS

- Do not use massage if your back pain is due to a fall or other injury or over an inflamed area.
- Stop the massage immediately if it is painful.
- Massage should not be done on the abdomen of pregnant women, or on those who have circulatory problems.
- Do not use any massage device without consulting your doctor.

TENS

Electrical therapy for pain relief is not a new concept. The ancient Greeks and Egyptians used electric eels, catfish and torpedo rays to produce analgesia. But the therapy was not widely accepted until Melzack and Wall formulated the gate control theory of pain (see page 28).

TENS (transcutaneous electric nerve stimulation) is a safe, convenient type of pain therapy. It utilizes low-voltage electricity to relieve pain by applying electrodes at acupuncture points to block the passage of pain sensations and stimulate the production of endorphins – the body's natural pain-relieving chemicals.

TENS is easy to learn and can be used in the course of daily activities as often as you wish. It is possible to buy a TENS machine through a physiotherapist or by mail order. But if you want to try one out first they can be hired, for use during labour for example, from local pharmacies and some mail-order companies.

CAUTION

- TENS seems to be contraindicated only in those people fitted with certain cardiac pacemakers. Check with your doctor before use.

ultrasound

Used by physiotherapists to treat various aches and pains, ultrasound utilizes sound waves of a frequency that is too high for the human ear to detect. It has three effects on the tissues:

- Its **mechanical** effect is that of a very fast mini-massage. In addition to improving circulation and drainage, reducing swelling and promoting relaxation, it can also accelerate the disintegration of small pieces of bone and grit in the joints.

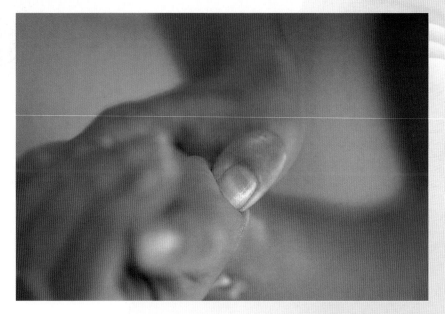

- Its **chemical** effect lies in the increase in the permeability of membranes to facilitate delivery of nutrients. It also dilates small blood vessels and helps to speed up the reduction of swelling.
- Its **thermal** (heat) effect improves circulation and promotes relaxation.

CAUTIONS
- Do not use ultrasound to treat aches and pains if you are pregnant.
- Ultrasound may make inflammation worse. Do not use it if you have an acute inflammatory condition or a blood disorder such as thrombosis or haemophilia.
- Do not use it over your eyes or heart, or over tumours, whether they are benign or malignant.

An acupressure practitioner applies pressure to energy points in order to encourage the body to return to a healthy state.

acupuncture and acupressure

These ancient forms of Oriental medicine date back 2,000 years or more. Both treatment types aim to balance the 'chi', or flow of energy, by working with points located along the body's energy channels, which are known as meridians.

Chinese medicine considers the state of health a result of the conflicting male and female forces of nature, termed 'yin' and 'yang'. When these forces are not in harmony, 'disease' ensues. A deficiency of chi results in pain.

An acupuncturist inserts fine sterile needles into particular acupuncture or energy points in order to balance energy flow, modify pain, influence disease states and also promote health and wellbeing.

In acupressure, the practitioner applies pressure to the same points to encourage the body to return to a healthy state.

Alexander Technique

The Alexander Technique teaches you how to remedy poor posture and use your body more safely and efficiently. You can read more about it on page 55.

chiropractic

Chiropractors use various examinations and manipulations to treat joint problems, in order to relieve pain and improve mobility and function.

Chiropractic was founded towards the end of the eighteenth century by a Canadian named Daniel David Palmer. It is based on the principle that the body's functions are controlled by the nervous system. Since this system is integrated with the body's musculoskeletal system, any disruptions in either one will affect the functioning of both. The aim of chiropractic treatment is to restore the balance and alignment of the whole structure.

Chiropractors place great importance on the spine and believe that even a minor spinal displacement will affect the nervous system. Their treatment often includes advice on proper body mechanics, for example, how to bend and lift correctly, and also preventive and corrective exercises to perform.

osteopathy

The practice of osteopathy dates back to the 1870s when the physician Andrew Taylor Still discovered the healing benefits of manual therapy. The main concept underlying this approach is that, given the best possible environment, the body can heal itself and restore natural balance.

Examination of the spine and joints forms the foundation of treatment. Osteopaths believe that since all body structures receive their nerve supply from the spinal cord, a spinal column that is not functioning optimally will generate problems. Manipulation of the back is a major part of their repertoire but they also work on the soft tissues around the spine.

relaxation

Relaxation is the common denominator of virtually all therapies aimed at pain relief. It decreases the activity of the sympathetic nervous system (which gears you up for activity such as 'fight' or 'flight') and activates the parasympathetic nervous system, which controls resting activities.

All Relaxation techniques (including Progressive Relaxation, pages 76–77) may be used as an adjunct to other procedures and therapies to enhance their pain-relieving effects.

biofeedback

The word 'biofeedback' refers to a method of training through which a person is able to influence certain body processes that were formerly thought to be beyond voluntary control. In biofeedback training, electrodes are attached to the subject's skin to pick up physiological signals such as blood pressure, pulse rate, body temperature, muscle tension or brain activity, which are then displayed as audio and video signals (sounds, coloured lights and meter readings). At the same time, the subject uses any one of a variety of relaxation techniques in order to gain control of the processes that are being monitored.

Biofeedback appeals to many patients as it helps them to feel some control over their healing. It is especially useful in stress-related conditions and spasmodic types of pain. It is often used in conjunction with visualization (see opposite). Once you have learned to relax using biofeedback techniques, you can dispense with the machine-monitoring and rely upon breathing exercises, visualization or some form of meditation instead.

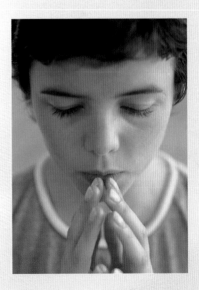

Meditation, visualization, imagery or conscious breathing can be practised without biofeedback to promote deep relaxation and so ease pain.

visualization and imagery

Visualization is the ability to create pictures in your mind. It is not merely wishful thinking nor is it a form of daydreaming or fantasizing, both of which are passive and unfocused. Visualization is active and purposeful.

When you visualize certain changes you wish to take place in your body, they tend to occur, even though you may be unaware of the underlying mechanisms. In some of the exercises (see pages 64–105), particularly those based on yoga and Pilates, visualization is encouraged to enhance their effectiveness.

Imagery is a flow of thoughts and includes sensory qualities from one or more of the senses, including smell, touch, hearing and taste, in addition to visualization. Imagery is commonly used in several body–mind therapies, including biofeedback as well as progressive muscle relaxation. It is also sometimes used to prepare patients for medical procedures and to relieve anxiety and pain.

Below is an exercise in visualization that you can do when experiencing pain or any other difficult sensation or emotion.

a healing visualization

1 Sit or lie comfortably and observe good posture. Relax your jaw and breathe regularly through your nose, but while inhaling pretend to be breathing through your mouth. You can close your eyes or keep them open if you prefer.

2 Rest your hands (or hand) lightly on the painful area or the part of the body where you feel the uncomfortable sensation most. As you take a slow, smooth breath inwards, visualize a soothing jet of warm water flowing along your arm to your hand and through your fingers into the affected part. Imagine that the water has healing properties.

3 As you breathe out slowly and smoothly, visualize a washing-away of irritants and impurities from the affected part; visualize them leaving your body on the outgoing breath.

4 Repeat steps 2 and 3 again and again in smooth succession, until you sense relief from your discomfort or pain.

5 Relax your arms and hands. Breathe regularly and steadily.

NOTES

You may modify this technique to breathe away fatigue, anger, frustration, resentment or other difficult emotion or sensation. Use imagery with which you feel absolutely comfortable. The above is a suggestion only.

breathing

The ancient practitioners of yoga were probably the first to discover the close relationship between breathing and mental states. This link has now been substantiated, and today breath is commonly used as a tool in healing therapies and other pain management approaches.

Changes in our feelings, especially if they are intense, are reflected in our patterns of breathing. When we are anxious, for example, our breathing tends to be faster than usual and sometimes irregular. But because our respiratory system is the only one that is both voluntary and involuntary, we can exercise a certain amount of control over it and influence the way we breathe. We can wilfully slow down our breathing to promote relaxation and calm.

In the exercises offered in this book, you will note that a great deal of emphasis is placed on breathing and on synchronizing movement with breathing. This is to encourage an awareness of the breath, our handiest tool for reducing tension build-up and stress, promoting muscle relaxation and coping with pain.

Breath supports many of our daily activities, and it is through the breath that oxygen is delivered to the working muscles. About

80 per cent of the work of breathing is accomplished by the diaphragm, which is a sheet of muscle located between the chest and the abdominal cavities. Poor use of the diaphragm in breathing is possibly at the root of a large number of health disorders. Diaphragmatic breathing is the most efficient way to breathe, as it uses a minimum of effort in return for a maximum intake of oxygen.

In addition to Rhythmic Diaphragmatic Breathing (pages 78–79), you will find the following two breathing exercises useful in helping you to cope with back pain and the anxiety that often accompanies and/or aggravates it.

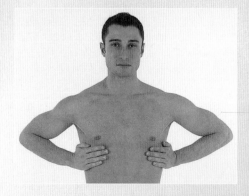

Diaphragmatic breathing, which uses a minimum of effort for a maximum intake of oxygen, is the most efficient way to breathe.

anti-anxiety breath

If your back pain is causing you anxiety or even a sense of panic, especially if you notice that you are not breathing normally, try this exercise to calm yourself down.

1 Sit tall, with the crown of your head uppermost. (You may also stand or lie down instead if you wish.) Relax your jaw and breathe regularly. Close your eyes, or keep them open if you prefer.

2 Inhale slowly, smoothly and as deeply as you can without strain, breathing in through your nose. Do not force yourself to take a deeper breath than you feel comfortable with.

3 Exhale through your nose as slowly, smoothly and completely as you can without force, and focusing your attention on your abdomen, near your navel.

4 Before inhaling again, mentally count 'one, one thousand', 'two, one thousand', to prolong your exhalation and prevent hyperventilation (overbreathing).

5 Repeat steps 2 to 4 again and again in smooth succession, until your breathing is slower and you feel calm.

6 Resume regular breathing and relax for a few minutes.

divided breath

When your chest feels so tight that you are unable to take a deep inward breath, this breathing exercise is the one to do to conquer the problem. Practise it any time you feel stressed, to help you to relax and regain control.

1 Sit or stand tall, with the crown of your head uppermost. (You may lie down instead if you wish.) Relax your jaw to facilitate breathing.

2 Take two or more fairly quick inward sniffs in succession, as if breaking up an inhalation into separate small parts.

3 Exhale slowly and steadily either through your nose, or through loosely pursed lips (as if you are whistling or blowing gently on a hot drink to cool it down).

4 Repeat steps 2 and 3 several times as necessary, until you feel that your chest is relaxing and that you can then take one deep inward breath without straining to do so.

5 Resume your regular breathing pattern and then relax for a short period.

rest positions

Although back pain sometimes responds well to a short period of bed rest, current wisdom is that keeping mobile is best for your back. Regular activity keeps the muscles that support the back strong and the spinal joints freely moving. The stronger and more flexible these structures are, the less vulnerable they will be to injury.

lying down

In general it is best to avoid lying face down as it subjects your lower back to unnecessary strain. When you do have to lie prone, however, place a thin pillow, cushion or folded towel under your hips. This will prevent an exaggeration of the spinal arch at the small of the back and reduce tension in the back muscles.

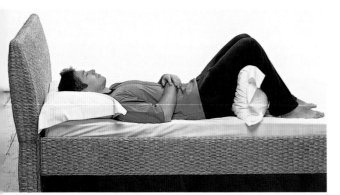

bed rest

In general, you should stay in bed for no more than a couple of days. Prolonged bed rest tends to weaken the back muscles and so aggravates existing back problems. It also accelerates bone loss and weakens discs and cartilage. When you rest in bed, do not sit up to read as sitting subjects your spine to further pressure.

PROGRESSIVE RELAXATION

Edmund Jacobson MD is credited with having devised the technique known as Progressive Relaxation in the 1920s. Practitioners of yoga, however, were already familiar with it many hundreds of years before. They called it Savasana in Sanskrit, which may be interpreted as the Pose of Tranquillity. Progressive Relaxation trains people to relax individual muscle groups in progression, until the whole body has achieved a state of deep relaxation. You will find detailed instructions for performing this relaxation technique in the section on cooling down and recovery on pages 76–77.

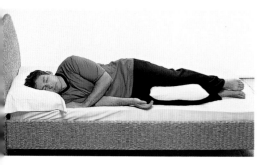

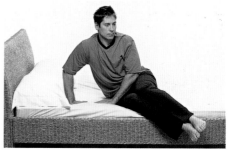

lying on your side

Lying on your side, with hip and knee joints bent, and pillows placed under the head and between bony prominences such as the knees, is one possible rest position. You should also lie on a firm supporting surface.

getting up

When you have been lying on your back, avoid sitting straight up. Instead, roll on to your side, bend your knees, bring them closer to your chest and use your hands to help push you on to your hip. Carefully pivot yourself until you are sitting evenly on your bottom, then slowly stand up. Breathe regularly throughout.

lying on your back

Another position that relaxes back muscles and promotes comfort is lying on the floor, on a non-skid mat or carpeted area, with your feet resting on a chair, bed or other suitable prop. Bend your knees to form a 90-degree angle and use a small pillow or rolled-up towel to support your neck. When preparing to lie in this position, carefully lift your legs one at a time.

Alternatively, you may find it comfortable to recline on a firm sofa, with your head and back supported, and a bolster or two or three pillows placed under your knees.

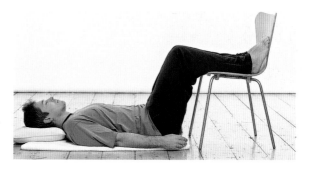

KEEPING MOBILE

Even during a period of bed rest, you should try getting up (using a proper technique, such as that described above) about every three hours, and moving around for around 20 to 30 minutes or as tolerated. Walk slowly and breathe regularly. Hold on to a counter, hand-rail or other stable prop for support, if necessary.

self-help for pain

When the first niggles of back pain creep up on you, you may decide to tackle the problem yourself – using one or more self-help techniques – before seeking help from your doctor or other health care professionals. If you have decided to treat your backache or back pain at home, here are some tips you may find helpful.

- Don't panic. Becoming upset will increase muscle tension and also aggravate the discomfort or pain.
- Stop and rest. Take a break from whatever you are doing and get off your feet. Use one of the rest positions described on pages 40–41. Avoid sitting, since it imposes a great deal of pressure on your spine.
- Lengthy rest periods, however, can weaken muscles. Try to get up (using the correct technique; see page 41) periodically and move around slowly for a few minutes every hour or so. If you can, do a few gentle stretches, in synchronization with your regular breathing.

- Try applying cold or heat to the painful area, observing the required precautions (see page 31).
- If possible, persuade someone to give you a gentle massage. When resting, practise a relaxation technique, such as that described on pages 36–37.
- If necessary, take a pain-relieving medicine, following all precautions as to dosage, frequency and interaction with other medicines.

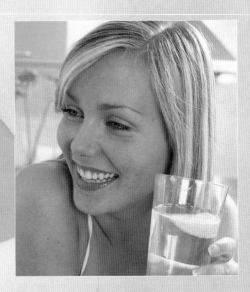

Dehydration exacerbates pain perception, so making sure you drink enough fluids to keep you fully hydrated is a simple and easy measure to take on board.

- Gradually resume your activities, but do so mindfully. Be conscious of your posture, either when still or when engaged in any activity.
- Avoid prolonged standing.
- Avoid driving for a while.
- Sleep on a firm surface.
- Drink plenty of fluids (particularly water) and eat lightly from a variety of wholesome foods.
- Consider making an appointment to see your doctor soon.

treating chronic pain

Pain that persists for over 12 weeks and does not respond to simple relief measures, such as brief periods of rest, often requires some type of pain-relieving medication. But you should be prudent in using these to avoid dependence on them.

Self-help measures include adherence to good postural habits and gentle stretching and strengthening exercises done regularly. Warming up prior to engaging in more strenuous tasks such as gardening or home improvement is essential. Other precautions include not wearing high-heeled shoes and not carrying a wallet or purse in your back pocket, as it may press on the sciatic nerve when you sit or drive.

Daily practice of some type of relaxation technique is also recommended as part of an essential stress-reduction programme. It is also important to eat well, choosing a wide variety of foods to help you get all the essential minerals and vitamins, and avoid foods that contribute to unnecessary weight gain.

If you have a chronic back problem, your doctor may refer you to a physiotherapist who may use one of the many methods available to ease your discomfort. Included in this repertoire are exercises to increase muscle strength and range of motion, and corrective exercises to improve posture and function. Other options include treatment by a chiropractor or an osteopath.

EMERGENCY MEASURES

If you have any of the following symptoms or signs, you should seek urgent medical care immediately. Do not delay in seeing a doctor if:

- your pain appears immediately or soon after you have lifted a heavy object (especially if you are older)
- your pain follows a recent minor injury, if you are over 60 years of age, particularly if you have osteoporosis
- your pain follows a blow (impact injury), fall or other accident
- you experience any numbness, weakness or swelling in your legs, feet, groin or rectum
- you are experiencing bladder or bowel problems (such as increased frequency of or difficulty in urination)
- your pain does not improve when you change position
- you have a fever or chills.

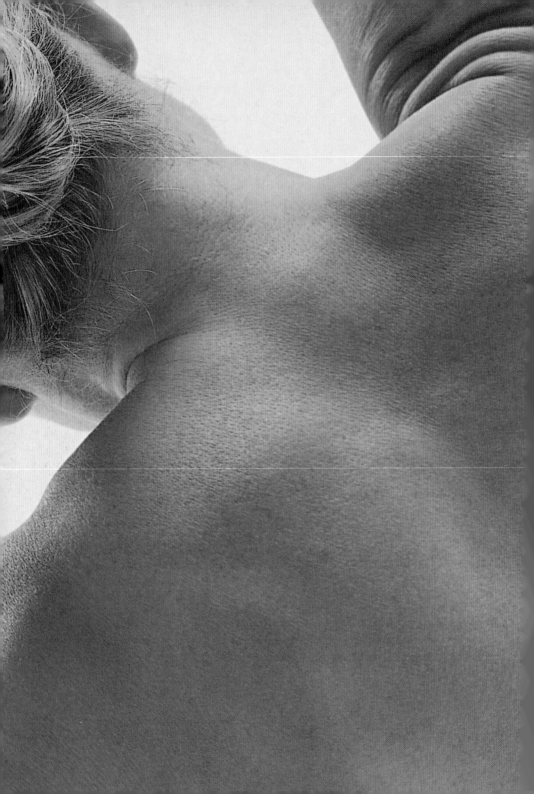

prevention is better than cure

You can do a great deal, perhaps more than you thought, to prevent back problems from arising in the first place. One very important step you can take is to do some form of stretching and strengthening exercise every day. If you are very busy, as so many people are, you can integrate exercises into your daily activities at work, at home or elsewhere. Another constructive step you can take towards attaining and maintaining a strong, flexible back, and so prevent some largely avoidable difficulties, is to get into the habit of practising good posture at all times.

body mechanics

Posture refers to the position of your body in space, regardless of whether you are sitting, standing, walking or lying down. Posture influences every aspect of your musculoskeletal system (the body's muscles and bony framework), and faulty posture is implicated in virtually every painful condition.

Body mechanics is a term used to refer to the way in which we use our body and its parts as we carry out various activities. Good posture and body mechanics require you to hold your body in such a way that your spine is well aligned, your muscles are not unduly tense or overstretched, and pressure on joints is even and natural. Anything else imposes unnecessary stress and is potentially damaging to the back and its related structures.

Cultivating good postural habits and practising good body mechanics are invaluable. The benefits include: reduced physical and emotional stress, fewer chances of developing back problems, easier breathing as well as an enhanced feeling of self-confidence.

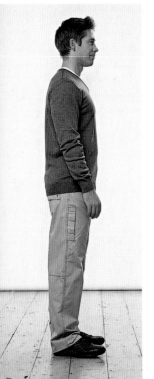

checking your posture

Standing in front of a full-length mirror, check the following points:

- Your head is level with the crown uppermost, and your chin is parallel to the floor.
- Your shoulders are directly below your ears and are level.
- Your hips are level.
- Your kneecaps point straight ahead and your knees are not locked.
- Your hands are relaxed and fall slightly in front of your thighs.

sitting

When you sit properly, your pelvis is in a neutral position: tilting neither backwards nor forwards. Folding your legs provides stability and encourages erect and relaxed back muscles.

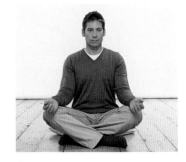

posture at work

If you spend many hours sitting at a desk, there are a few simple measures you can take to prevent back ailments. When seated, you should ideally be able to:

- Place your feet flat on the floor or on a foot rest.
- Have your lower back supported.
- Maintain about a 90-degree (or slightly greater) angle between your thighs and your back.
- Keep your forearms, wrists and hands in a straight line.
- View your computer screen slightly below eye level.

Here are additional tips to help ensure a trouble-free back at work:

- Do not cross your legs. It tilts the pelvis too far forwards, increases the spinal curve at the small of the back and subjects the back to even greater strain.
- Organize your work area so that all the items you regularly need are within easy reach, and others are accessible with a minimum of bending and reaching.
- Do not cradle your telephone handset between your ear and your shoulder. Use a headset or speaker phone instead if this is possible.
- Do not bite on your pen or pencil or chew on hard items like ice. This stresses your jaw joints and muscles. Unclench your teeth to keep your jaw relaxed.
- Keep well hydrated by drinking water periodically.

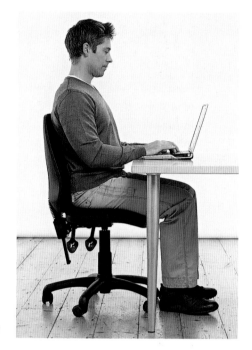

driving

Even if your job does not require driving long distances, you probably still spend many hours driving a car or other motor vehicle during the course of a week. To reduce the chances of neck and back problems, here are some simple rules to follow:

- Make sure that your seat is adjusted so that your feet can comfortably reach the various pedals without them being locked straight.
- Use and adjust a well-designed headrest to protect your neck.
- Use a back support if necessary.
- Use a seat belt with both lap and chest components.
- Maintain good posture.

posture at play

Sports provide opportunities for enhancing the function of your muscles, tendons, ligaments and joints. They can also help to make you less vulnerable to stiffness, aches and soreness, and diminish your chances of developing such degenerative disorders of the musculoskeletal system as osteoarthritis.

But some sports pose an increased risk of injury, particularly if you are not in shape, or if you have not prepared yourself properly. Adequate warming up is crucial and flexibility exercises are also recommended, with emphasis on those areas of the body you use most in your chosen sport. Cooling down properly afterwards is also imperative.

For people who are inactive most of the week but engage in sports at the weekend, additional training may be required to build necessary strength, endurance and flexibility. It may also be prudent to consult a physical therapist or qualified trainer.

golf

Many golfers suffer from back problems. These are largely related to the twisting motion that accompanies the drive. If you are thinking of taking up golf, it is definitely a good idea to consider taking lessons to help you develop a good technique from the start. To lessen the chances of damage to spinal joints and the intervertebral discs, aim at developing a swing that minimizes twisting

motions. Also consider wearing non-spiked shoes to reduce impact at the end of the swing.

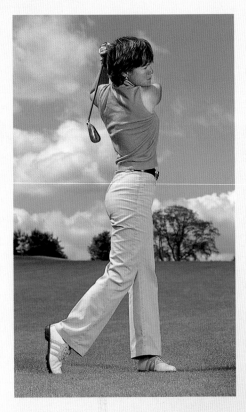

Master your golf swing with professional coaching so that you don't get into bad postural habits or twist awkwardly when playing a round or two.

downhill skiing

The increased muscle tension from poor posture while skiing can be damaging to your back. Concentrate on maintaining good posture and lengthen your torso as you bend your knees. Keep your hip joints loose so you can comfortably rotate back and forth as you travel downhill.

Remember to warm up properly before skiing, and to also include a full body stretch in your pre-ski exercise routine.

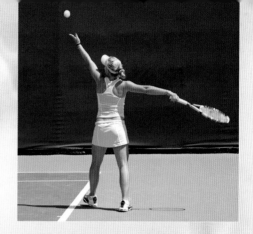

To meet the demands of tennis, be sure to keep your torso lengthened, knee and hip joints loose and your body as relaxed as possible.

tennis

Racquet sports, such as tennis, can add force to the actions of bending and twisting and so precipitate a number of back ailments. Avoid hunching over from your waist or shoulders as you play. Lengthen your body upwards and think of your racquet as an extension of your arm. Avoid twisting your torso when you reach for the ball. If necessary, take lessons to learn a proper technique.

Warm up slowly and sufficiently before playing, and include a full body stretch to avoid straining muscles.

posture en route

If you travel frequently by air, here is an exercise to prevent a sore back. Do it while waiting to board an aircraft and also periodically in flight. It is a sitting version of the Pelvic Tilt (see page 93).

1 Inhale through your nose, slowly and smoothly.

2 As you exhale slowly and smoothly, press the small of your back (at waist level) towards or against the back of your seat. Maintain this pressure for as long as your exhalation.

3 Inhale through your nose and relax your back.

4 Repeat steps 2 and 3 several times. Relax and rest.

Keep your lower back supported with a small cushion. You may find a modified version of the Chest Expansion exercise (see page 80) helpful in reducing tension in your upper back. Squeeze your shoulder blades together as you inhale, and relax your upper back and shoulders as you exhale.

daily activities

During our activities of daily living we can inadvertently develop certain postural habits that, with repetition, feel right. Just because they are comfortable, however, does not mean that they are safe. Over time, they may, in fact, put our back at risk by subjecting it to unnecessary stress and wear and tear.

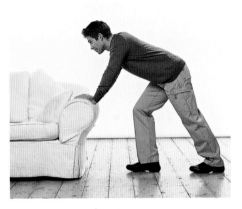

pulling or pushing

When you have to shift heavy objects such as items of furniture or a loaded wheelbarrow, avoid pulling them. Whenever possible, use a pushing action, keeping your knees slightly bent and your neck and back in the correct alignment.

carrying heavy loads

If you can, divide a heavy load into several lighter ones, even if it means making extra trips. If the load cannot be divided, ask someone to help you carry it, or use a trolley. If no help is available, and you need to carry the load in your arms, be sure to hold it close to your body.

Avoid carrying weight on only one side of your body, such as a single bag of groceries or a large flight bag. If possible, divide it into two lighter bags and carry one in each hand.

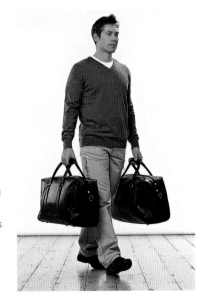

comfortable sexual positions

You do not have to forgo an enjoyable and active sex life if you have back problems, unless, that is, you are experiencing muscle spasm or acute back pain. The physical activity of intercourse may, in fact, be beneficial, provided that you use positions that are easy on your back. In most cases a little experimentation with different positions and the use of pillows will make sexual activity fun and pain-free again.

Some positions that are easy on your back and that may work for you include the following:

- Lying on your side facing your partner.
- Lying on your side with hips and knees bent, facing the same direction as your partner. This 'spoons' arrangement is great if you both suffer from back ailments.
- The partner with the back problem on top, with knees bent. The partner

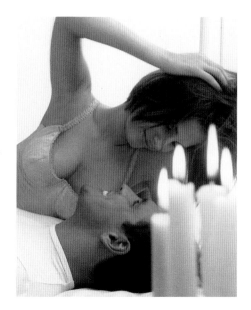

Try out a few sexual positions to find one that is pain-free and works for both of you.

below propped up with extra pillows. This tilts the pelvis and helps to minimize stress on the lower back.

twisting movements

A common cause of strain or spasm of back muscles or of intervertebral disc problems is any sudden twisting of the trunk, as can happen when you are picking up or reaching for an object or moving something from one place to another and you are moving only the top of your body.

In these instances, such as transferring clean laundry from a washing machine to an adjacent tumble dryer, you should move your

feet, turn your whole body and bend your knees rather than just twisting your upper body, to protect your back.

Although it is an instinctive reaction, avoid any sudden attempt to catch a falling object. Your muscles may not have sufficient time to contract properly to protect the spinal joints. Also, the contractions may not be perfectly coordinated, and damage to muscles and ligaments may result.

lifting know-how

Whenever you lift something heavy – a storage box, a piece of furniture or a child, for example – avoid rounding your back and be sure to bend from your knees so that your leg muscles take the strain. Then, when you set the object down, repeat the sequence in reverse.

to lift a box

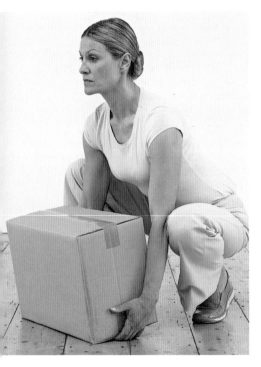

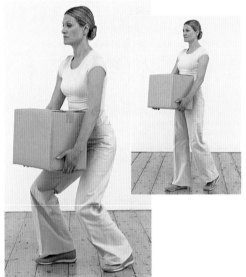

1 Keeping your back straight, squat down with one foot slightly in front of the other and with the box between your knees. Grasp the box from underneath with both hands and straighten your arms.

2 Lean forwards slightly, still keeping your back straight. Holding the box close to your body, stand up straight, in a controlled way, taking the weight on your legs. Keep the box close to your body while you carry it.

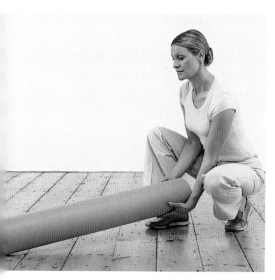

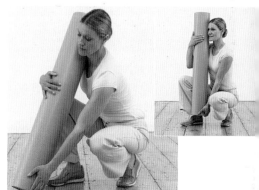

1 Squat down with one leg slightly in front of the other and one end of the load between your feet. Keeping your back straight, place your hands around the nearer end.

2 Slowly ease the load into a vertical position, then lift it against your shoulder, using one hand to support the bottom and placing your other hand further up to steady it.

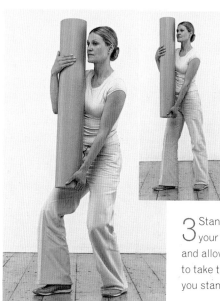

3 Stand up, keeping your back straight and allowing your legs to take the weight, as you stand up.

best remedy

The consensus of experts on back care is that most problems can be satisfactorily controlled by a combination of non-surgical treatments. These include physiotherapy, exercise and medications. Whatever the combination may be, the one factor that appears again and again – whether it is to prevent difficulties, to maintain function or for rehabilitation following trauma or surgery – is exercise. There are very good reasons for this.

benefits of exercise

Regular, appropriate exercise improves the strength of the muscles supporting the back. It also keeps the joints moving freely. The stronger and more flexible these structures are, the less vulnerable they will be to potentially damaging forces.

Regular exercise also helps to prevent or delay the onset of osteoporosis, which makes spinal and other bones more prone to fracture. Stretching exercises facilitate the removal of wastes, such as lactic acid (which is associated with fatigue), from the muscles. Regular exercise, moreover, helps you to cope with stress and so reduces your chances of becoming anxious, a state that aggravates pain.

Exercise has a place in the physical treatment of even the most painful of musculoskeletal conditions, as an adjunct to other treatments. This is partly because it appears to increase endorphin levels. Exercise is also an antidote to sleeplessness, which many back pain sufferers often experience.

Before proceeding with the exercises themselves, and with the requisite guidelines and cautions, let's look at the chief approaches on which they are based.

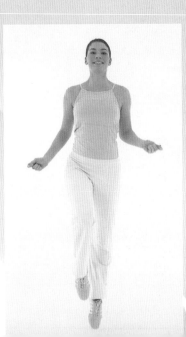

Whether it's to prevent back problems or to restore function after an injury, regular exercise is essential.

Alexander Technique

This technique teaches you how to use your body correctly during your daily activities and so to eliminate poor postural habits. Adhering to the Alexander Technique will help to prevent the accumulation of the muscular tension that aggravates fatigue, aches, pain and other physiological disorders.

The technique was developed towards the end of the nineteenth century by Frederick Matthias Alexander, an Australian actor. He was plagued by a chronic hoarseness (especially when he was on stage) that did not respond well to any conventional medical treatments, so he embarked on a journey of meticulous self-observation and behavioural changes. Eventually these brought him the improvements he was looking for and helped him develop an organized method for the control and change of the physical and behavioural habits that were at the root of his difficulties.

The main objective of the technique is to encourage people to use their body and mind more efficiently in day-to-day living. This is referred to as 'good use', which involves less stressful ways of sitting, standing and walking. Teachers of the Alexander Technique attempt to establish a relationship with their students that is based on trust. Their aim is to encourage in the student an understanding of the essential principles of the technique. They point out that poor postural habits, or what they call 'misuse', can cause strain in these areas and so generate pain and various ailments. Alexander Technique teachers use their hands to move the student into the correct posture and also give verbal instructions and explanations as part of their therapy. The Alexander Technique is respected by health care professionals. Among its main uses it can help to relieve musculoskeletal problems, cumulative stress injuries and back pain.

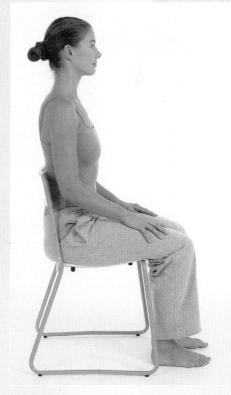

An important principle of the Alexander Technique is the awareness of posture and patterns of movement. The key to this is the coordination of the head, neck and back.

Pilates

Named after its creator, Joseph H. Pilates, this system of exercises combines the best of Western and Eastern traditions, encouraging an awareness of body and mind working together in harmony.

Born in Germany in 1880, Pilates was very sickly as a child but as he grew older he was determined to make himself stronger, becoming proficient in body-building and gymnastics. After emigrating to the USA in 1926, Pilates opened a studio in New York where he taught an approach to fitness he called 'Contrology'. It was not long before he had an enthusiastic following, particularly among athletes, dancers and actors.

Today, Pilates' method is enjoying a surge of popularity worldwide, not only among the general public but also among various professionals – athletes, dancers and health care professionals. Because Pilates emphasizes strengthening the 'powerhouse' – the muscles between the rib cage and the hips – it is particularly useful in helping to prevent back problems.

Swiss ball

The Swiss ball (also known as an exercise, physio or stability ball) was developed in the 1900s to treat neurological disorders such as spinal cord injuries and stroke. Not long afterwards, fitness professionals began to use it as an exercise tool in order to help improve balance and strengthen postural muscles (of the abdomen, back and legs).

The benefit of the ball lies in its instability: your muscles have to work to keep it stable during exercise movements, mainly those muscles of the abdomen and lower back.

Available in various sizes to suit every age, height and level of ability, exercise balls are usually made of a durable vinyl. The choice of ball generally depends on the exercise method being used. With Pilates-based work, for example, a 55 cm (22 in) ball generally works well, unless you are very tall and fit.

A good tip to help you select the right exercise ball for your size is that when you sit on the ball with your feet flat on the floor, your thighs should be parallel to the floor and the angle of

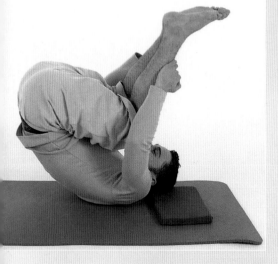

The key to the effectiveness of Pilates in easing back pain is the focus given to building strength in the torso.

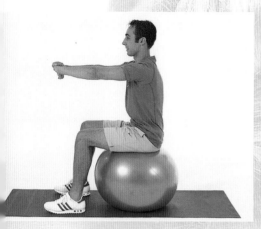

Strengthen your postural muscles by working out with the Swiss ball – keeping it steady is part of the fun.

than four thousand years, it continues to enjoy tremendous popularity worldwide, and is now the basis of many other stress-reduction and health-promotion programmes.

Hatha Yoga is the form most commonly practised in Western countries. Its primary goal is to prevent health disorders and promote general wellbeing but, if illness does arise, it assists those who practise it regularly to regain and maintain optimum health. It does this through a balanced system of non-strenuous stretching and strengthening 'physical' exercises ('asanas'), breathing techniques ('pranayama') and also various relaxation and meditative exercises.

Emphasis is also placed on correct posture and spinal health, and awareness in all movement and action – a sort of fine tuning that is useful in preventing accidental injury.

both your hip and your knee joints should be 90 degrees. As a general rule, a ball of 55 cm (22 in) in diameter is suitable for people between 152 cm (5 ft) and 173 cm (5 ft 8 in) tall and a 65 cm (26 in) ball would suit those people who are between 173 cm (5 ft 8 in) and 188 cm (6 ft 2 in) tall.

yoga

The word 'yoga' comes from the Sanskrit language and means 'to integrate'. It is an approach to health care that promotes the harmonious working together of all the body's components.

Because of its roots in the Hindu culture of India, some people erroneously believe that yoga is a religion. In fact yoga is non-sectarian and can be practised by anyone. Although yoga has existed for more

Smooth stretching done with awareness, synchronized with slow breathing are characteristic of yoga exercises.

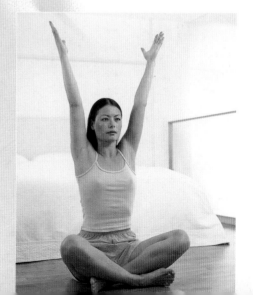

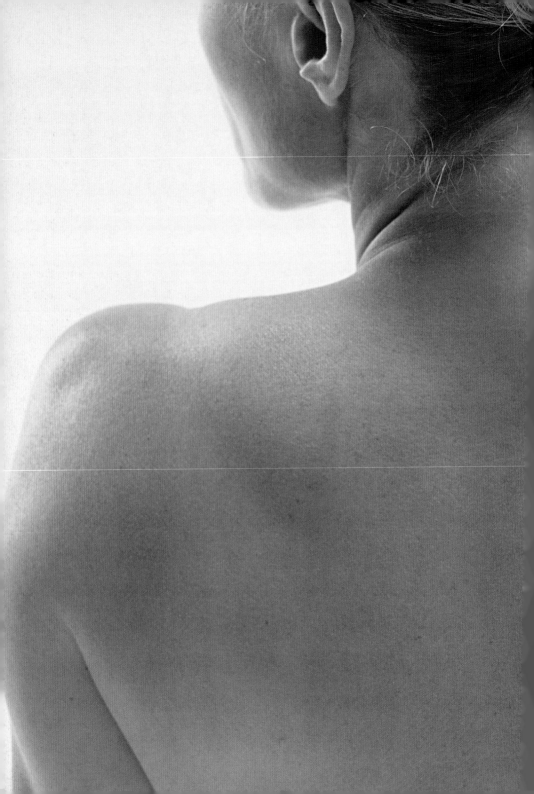

exercises
for a
better back

Now that you understand how your back works
and how to take care of it in theory, it is time to
put that knowledge into action. Before you launch into
the exercises that follow, however, read the guidelines and
cautions carefully. Make sure that you always warm up
before you start and allow time to cool down gradually
afterwards. The main exercises begin on page 80
and the suggested programmes on page 108.

guidelines

The following general guidelines are designed to help you incorporate an exercise programme into your daily schedule. Most experts on back care agree that the most effective way to prevent and treat back problems is through regular exercise. An enjoyable regular session combining exercise, attention to breathing and relaxation will keep your back flexible and toned, and will be your best insurance against back pain.

Before you start any programme of exercise it is important to consider your level of fitness so that you can start at an appropriate level. The exercises in this book are all graded as suitable for beginners or those at intermediate or advanced level.

warming-up

It is important to introduce yourself to any exercise programme gradually. Don't make the mistake of overdoing it and causing more damage than you had before.

The golden rule is always to allow some time to warm up before your main activity and to cool down afterwards. Warming up prepares the heart muscles for exercise and stretches the skeletal muscles. This helps to reduce stiffness and to prevent muscular pulls and strain. The exercises on pages 64–73 are especially suitable for warm ups, whereas those on pages 74–79 will help you to cool down and relax after you have completed the programme.

regular routine

Choose a time of day and a place where you will be able to complete a programme, including warming up and cooling down, without being distracted or disturbed by the phone or family, for example.

If it is possible, arrange to practise regularly and often – a 10-minute session every day or every other day is better than a single 30-minute session once a week. And if you can, try to get into the habit of doing your exercises at about the same time each day so that you learn to make them part of your daily routine – soon you'll do them without even thinking about it.

Also remember that it is often possible to incorporate certain exercises into your daily life. You could get into the habit of doing Neck Stretches (see page 65) during television advertising breaks, for example, doing a few Shoulder Circles (see page 66) while you are waiting for the kettle to boil or even at work secretly incorporate the Perineal Exercise (see page 17) into those boring office meetings.

comfort

For your regular exercise sessions it is best to wear comfortable clothing that permits ease of movement and breathing – but make sure it is warm enough. While you are doing cooling down exercises, you may need to have extra blankets, socks or a warm top nearby in case you feel chilled. Most of the exercises are best done barefoot so that you don't slip. Avoid exercising immediately after a meal or when you are very tired. And for comfort, remember to empty your bladder before a session.

safety

For safety, always practise on a non-slip surface. Also remember to remove any items such as glasses or jewellery that may cause pressure or injury or become uncomfortable. If exercising during breaks at work, loosen your clothing a little.

how to practise

The key words to guide your practice are: 'slowly', 'smoothly' and 'attentively'. It is important to concentrate on what you are doing and be aware of the effect it is having on your body. This will help to prevent injury caused by overexertion.

As you perform the steps of an exercise, synchronize your movements with regular breathing. This will facilitate the delivery of oxygen to working muscles and also help to maximize the exercise's beneficial effects. As discussed earlier, an awareness of breathing is central to reducing the build-up of stress and tension, which results in pain.

Don't forget to rest briefly for a few seconds between exercises to avoid stiffness and fatigue. After each set of exercise instructions, suggestions are given for the number of times to do the exercises and the number of seconds to hold (maintain) the completed position. These numbers are a minimum. Adjust them to suit your own circumstances and level of fitness. As you get fitter and stronger, you can add more repetitions.

visualizations

You may also find it helpful to use your visualization techniques to enhance the effectiveness of the exercises. Visualization and imagery tap into the powerful pain-relieving mechanisms you have at your disposal in your brain and nervous system.

equipment

If you are using an exercise ball, make sure you follow the manufacturer's instructions regarding its care and safe use. For example, some exercises using the ball require the use of footwear for safety.

If you use light weights while exercising, weights of 0.5 to 1.5 kg (1 to 3 lb) should suffice. Do not use weights that are heavier than 2.5 kg (5 lb).

taking care

Before attempting to do any of the exercises in this book, or indeed starting any exercise programme, it is advisable to check with your doctor that what you plan to do is appropriate. This is especially important if you have had surgery, if you have osteoporosis, arthritis or a spinal problem or if you are pregnant.

cautions in pregnancy

Many physical instructors generally advise against starting Pilates-based exercises, such as those listed below, during the early stages of pregnancy, that is during the first 12 weeks, or the first trimester. After that first precious time, Pilates is a great exercise for improving core strength.

- Rolling Like a Ball (page 72)
- Seal (page 73)
- Roll Down (pages 74–75)
- Pilates Spine Twist (page 83)
- Roll Up (pages 90–91)
- Teaser (modified) (pages 94–95)
- Swan Dive (pages 98–99)
- Rocking (page 100)
- Swimming (page 101)
- Dog Stretch (page 102)
- Single-Leg Kicks (page 103)

Check first with your doctor if you wish to do them while pregnant.

- Do not do the exercises in the first three or four months if you have a history of actual or threatened miscarriage (bleeding in the first 12 weeks).
- Omit exercises in the prone position (lying on the abdomen) in pregnancy, such as the Swan Dive (pages 98–99) and the Prone Leg Raise (page 101).
- Avoid doing any exercise that feels awkward or uncomfortable.

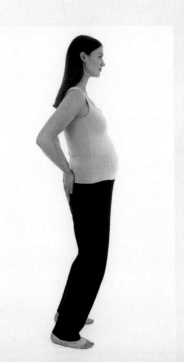

Good postural habits and a balance of regular, gentle exercise and rest will do much to control back pain during pregnancy.

- After 30 weeks, when your baby starts to get quite big, it's a good idea to avoid doing exercises that entail lying flat on your back. In this position, your baby can squash the major vein supplying the lower body, restricting blood flow and oxygen to mother and foetus.

general cautions

- Do not do any exercise that causes pain. If your back condition worsens, decrease your activity. Modify the exercises in this book to suit your own special needs.
- If you have a hernia or heart condition, avoid the Swan Dive (pages 98–99), the Prone Leg Raise (page 101) and the Rocking exercise (page 100).
- Omit the Seal (page 73) if you have problems with your neck.
- Avoid staying in the Squatting posture (page 105) if you have venous blood clots or varicose veins.
- Avoid sitting for a long period in a folded-legs posture (see page 82) if you have venous blood clots or varicose veins.
- Omit the Dog Stretch (page 102) if you suffer from high blood pressure, have a heart disorder or any condition that produces feelings of lightheadedness or dizziness when you hang your head down.
- If you have osteoporosis,

spondylolysis or spondylolisthesis, or have suffered a recent spinal fracture, avoid forward-bending postures as they may damage vertebrae or aggravate existing symptoms.
- Before engaging in vigorous activity or strenuous work in the morning, just after a night's sleep, do warm up properly.
- When resuming exercise after a period of inactivity, following illness for example, do so very gradually. Please consult your doctor, physiotherapist or other qualified health professional. If you have had recent surgery or are recovering from an injury, it is imperative that you follow the advice of your doctor or physiotherapist regarding exercise.
- Do review the first three sections of the book from time to time to remind yourself about the function and structure of the spine, the importance of posture and how to prevent back pain.

Before attempting any exercise programme consult your doctor. If you have a specific health problem, check the list of cautions for any exercise you should avoid.

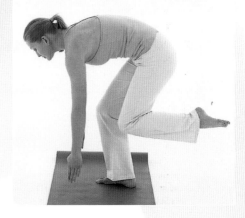

warm-ups

Warming up is a very important part of any exercise programme. Warm-ups help to reduce stiffness, slightly increase body temperature and improve blood and lymph circulation. They are also a preventive measure against muscular pulls and strains once the main exercises are in progress.

The following warm-up exercises have been carefully chosen with the health of the spine and its supports in mind. Several of them, such as the Neck Stretches (opposite) and the Shoulder Circles (see page 66), for example, can be integrated into daily activities (such as waiting for the kitchen timer to ring while you prepare a meal) to avert tension build up, which can generate fatigue and aches and pain in the back.

chin glide (turtle)

Strengthens the cervical spine. Wards off neck stiffness
Enhances the range of motion of the neck

Sit or stand tall, with the crown of your head uppermost, relax your shoulders. Relax your jaw and breathe regularly through your nose. As you exhale, slowly and smoothly thrust your chin forwards, like a turtle sticking out its neck. Inhale and slowly resume your starting position. Repeat the exercise and then rest.

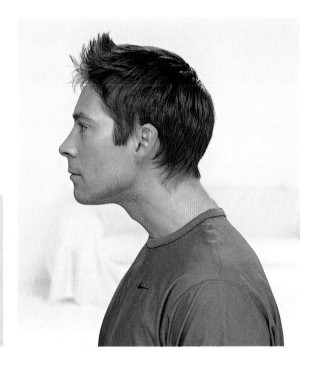

INTERMEDIATE
3 times, along with the other
   Neck Stretches
ADVANCED
3 times, along with the other
   Neck Stretches

neck stretch

Reduces stiffness and promotes flexibility of the neck
Prevents tension build-up in the neck
Improves circulation in the neck and surrounding structures

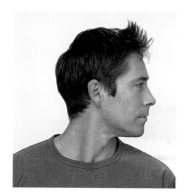

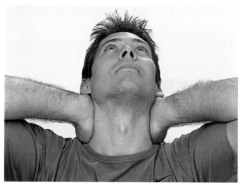

1 Sit or stand tall, with the crown of your head uppermost. Relax your shoulders. Relax your jaw and breathe regularly through your nose throughout the exercise. Turn your head to the left. Pause for a few seconds. Turn your head back to the middle. Turn your head to the right and pause for a few seconds. Turn your head back to the middle.

2 Support the back of your neck with your hands and carefully tilt your head backwards. Pause for a few seconds. Carefully bring your head upright and relax your arms and hands.

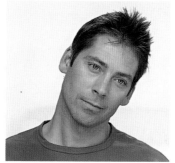

BEGINNER
3 times

INTERMEDIATE
3 times

ADVANCED
3 times

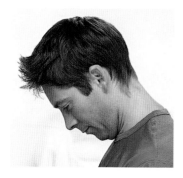

3 Carefully tilt your head forwards, aiming your chin to your chest. Pause for a few seconds. Bring your head upright.

4 Tilt your head to the left, aiming ear to shoulder. Pause briefly. Bring your head upright. Tilt your head to the right, aiming ear to shoulder. Pause briefly. Bring your head upright. Rest briefly. Repeat the series (steps 2 to 4) three times, resting briefly between each series.

shoulder circle

Reduces stiffness in the shoulders
Prevents the build-up of tension in shoulders and upper back
Enhances the effects of the Neck Stretches (see page 65)

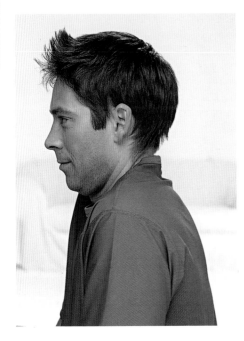

1 Sit or stand tall, with the crown of your head uppermost. Keep your arms loose and hands relaxed. Relax your jaw and breathe regularly through your nose while doing the exercises. Slowly and smoothly rotate both shoulders in a backwards-to-forwards motion, as if drawing imaginary circles with them. Rest briefly.

2 Repeat step 1, this time in a forwards-to-backwards motion. Relax and rest.

BEGINNER 6 times

INTERMEDIATE 6 times

ADVANCED 8 times

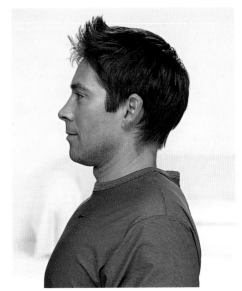

arm circle with weights

Keeps the shoulder joints moving freely
Strengthens the arms, shoulders and upper back
Helps build bone mass and so prevent osteoporosis

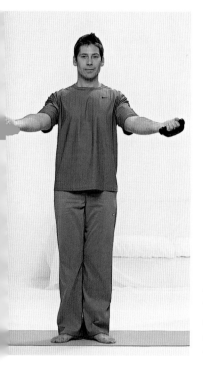

Stand tall, with the crown of your head uppermost, your heels together and toes pointing slightly outwards. Relax your jaw and breathe regularly through your nose during the exercise. Start with your arms down and a little away from your sides, and a 1–1.5 kg (2–3 lb) weight in each hand. Make small circles, slowly and smoothly, away from your body, as you gradually raise your arms to chest level or higher. Try to keep your arms to your sides or slightly to the front – whichever you find more comfortable. Slowly and smoothly make similar circles – this time towards your body – while gradually lowering your arms. Rest briefly. Repeat the exercise, circling your arms in the opposite direction.

BEGINNER 4 times

INTERMEDIATE 6 times

ADVANCED 8 times

foot circles

Keeps the ankle joints moving freely
Strengthens the feet
Improves circulation in the feet and legs

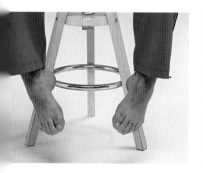

Sit where you can move your feet freely. Maintain good posture and breathe regularly through your nose while doing the exercise. Make circles with your feet: clockwise with one, and anticlockwise with the other. (Alternatively, rotate one ankle at a time.) Repeat the exercise in the opposite direction. Rest.

BEGINNER 6 times

INTERMEDIATE 6 times

ADVANCED 8 times

butterfly

Counteracts stiffness in the hip and ankle joints
Gently stretches and strengthens the inner thigh muscles
Improves circulation in the pelvic region

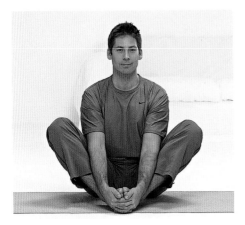 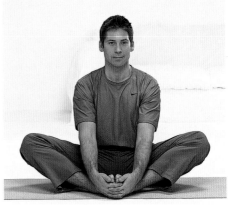

1 Sit tall on your mat, with your legs out straight in front of you. Relax your jaw and breathe regularly throughout the exercise. Fold your legs inwards, one at a time, to bring the soles of your feet together. Clasp your hands around your feet and bring them comfortably close to your body.

2 At a smooth and moderate pace, alternately lower and raise your knees, like a butterfly flapping its wings. Carefully stretch out your legs, one at a time. Relax your hands. Rest.

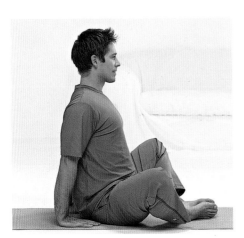

VARIATION

If you are a beginner, you will probably find it easier to support yourself by placing your hands just behind you with your palms flat on the mat rather than clasping your feet.

BEGINNER Variation, 20 times

INTERMEDIATE 30 times

ADVANCED 30 times

single-knee hug

Strengthens the muscles of the back and abdomen; the variation also strengthens the neck muscles
Relieves tiredness, strain and aching in the back
Keeps the spine flexible

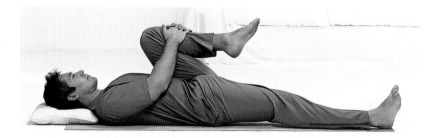

Lie on your back with your legs stretched out in front, and your arms at your sides. Breathe regularly through your nose. (If you wish, place a small pillow under your head.) Exhaling, slowly bring one bent leg towards your chest; keep the small of your back pressed to the mat. Hold your lower leg and maintain the position for a few seconds while breathing regularly. Release your hold on the bent leg and slowly lower it to the mat as you inhale. Rest while breathing regularly. Repeat the exercise with your other leg.

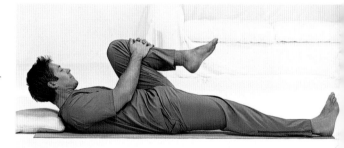

VARIATION

Follow the above. Hold the bent leg securely, then carefully lift your head as if to touch the bent knee. Maintain this position for a few seconds while breathing regularly. Carefully lower your head to the mat then lower your leg as you inhale. Repeat with the other leg.

BEGINNER
Knee to chest only, 4 times

INTERMEDIATE
Variation, 5 times

ADVANCED
Variation, 6 times

lying twist

Strengthens abdominal muscles
Strengthens lower back muscles
Keeps the lower back flexible

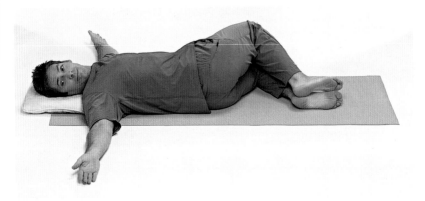

Lie on your back with your arms stretched out at shoulder level. Relax your jaw and breathe regularly through your nose. (If you wish, place a small pillow under your head.) Bend your legs, one at a time, then bring both knees up towards your chest. Keeping your arms and shoulders pressed to the mat, exhale and slowly tilt both knees to the side. You may keep your head still or turn it in the opposite direction to your knees. Inhale and bring your knees and head to the centre. Repeat, tilting your knees to the opposite side. Stretch out your legs, one at a time. Bring your arms to your sides and rest.

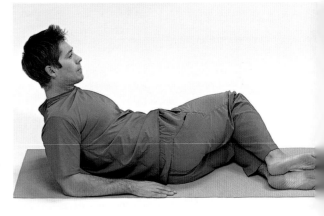

VARIATION

From a sitting position, lean back on your elbows. Bring your knees towards your chest, one at a time. Alternately tilt your knees towards the left and right, in synchronization with regular breathing. Stretch out and rest.

BEGINNER Variation, 6 times

INTERMEDIATE 8 times

ADVANCED 10 times

lying twist with ball

Strengthens inner thigh muscles
Strengthens abdominal and lower back muscles
Keeps the lower back flexible

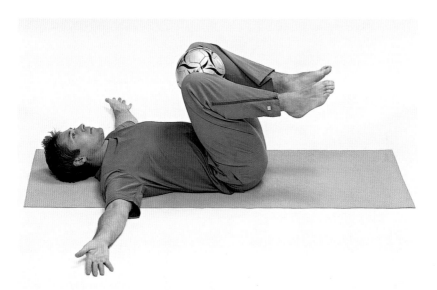

1 Lie on your back with your legs bent and the soles of your feet flat on the mat. Place a small exercise ball to fit securely between your knees. Stretch your arms sideways at shoulder level. Relax your jaw and breathe regularly through your nose. (You may rest your head on a small pillow.) Lift your feet to bring your bent knees, with the ball in between, towards your chest.

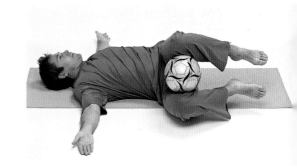

INTERMEDIATE 8 times

ADVANCED 10 times

2 Exhale and tilt your knees to one side. Inhale and bring your knees to the centre. Exhale and tilt your knees to the opposite side. Inhale and bring your knees to the centre. Rest.

rolling like a ball

Massages the back muscles
Strengthens the abdominal muscles
Gently stretches the hamstring muscles to help prevent shortening

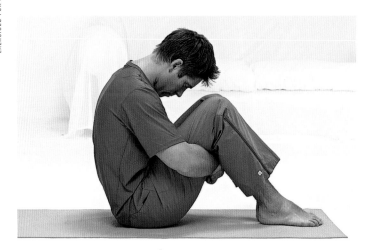

1 Sit tall on your mat. Bend your legs and rest the soles of your feet flat on the mat close to your bottom. Pass your hands under your knees and hug your thighs. Tuck your chin in. Make your back as rounded as you comfortably can. Relax your jaw and breathe regularly through your nose.

2 Inhale and kick backwards to help you roll on to your back. Exhale and rock forwards to bring you back into a sitting position. Do not land heavily on your feet to jar your spine. Repeat the exercise again and again in smooth succession. Rest.

INTERMEDIATE 8 times

seal

Massages the back muscles
Strengthens the abdominal muscles
Gently stretches the hamstring muscles to help prevent shortening

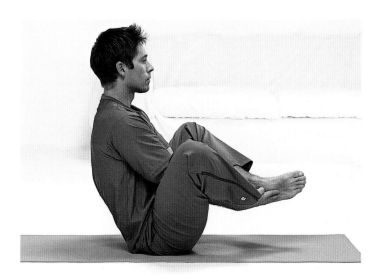

1 Sit tall on your mat. Bend your legs and rest the soles of your feet flat on the mat. Pass your hands between your legs and hold on to your ankles. Tuck your chin in. Relax your jaw and breathe regularly through your nose. Lift your feet off the mat with the soles together until you are balancing on your coccyx (tailbone).

2 Breathe in and roll backwards, at the same time clapping your heels together three times, just like a sea lion 'clapping' its flippers. Exhale and roll forwards. Again clap your heels together three times while balancing on your bottom. Repeat the exercise again and again in smooth succession. And, then, rest.

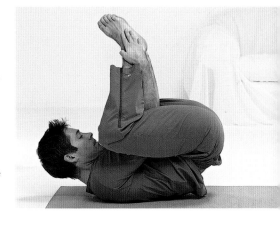

ADVANCED 6 to 8 times

cool down

It is as important to cool down after an exercise session as it is to warm up beforehand. Cooling down provides an opportunity for static muscle stretching, which enhances flexibility. It also allows your heart and blood vessels to return gradually to normal functioning and helps to prevent any sudden drops in blood pressure, feelings of lightheadedness and dizziness – any of which can occur if you stop exercising abruptly. A cool-down period protects you against extreme temperature changes in the lungs, which in some people (such as those with asthma) can exacerbate respiratory symptoms.

Done leisurely and attentively, all the warm-up exercises in this section (see pages 64–73) can also be used for cooling down, except the Arm Circles using weights, the Butterfly, Rolling Like a Ball and the Seal.

Here are four other exercises that you can do as part of your cool down and recovery routine.

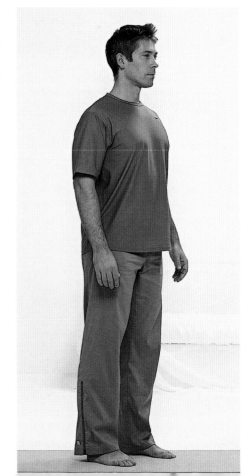

roll down

Counteracts body stiffness
Promotes relaxation
Replenishes energy reserves

1 Stand tall, with your arms at your sides. Relax your jaw and breathe regularly through your nose while doing this exercise.

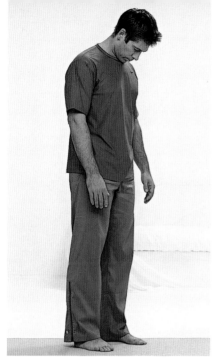

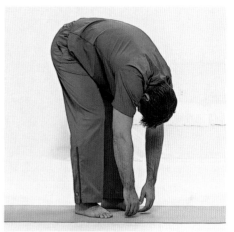

2 Slowly tilt your head to your chest. Let your shoulders droop and your arms and hands go limp.

3 Let the rest of your body curl forwards slowly and smoothly; feel the weight of your arms pulling you downwards until your body hangs loosely, with your arms dangling. Imagine being a floppy rag doll. Stay in this posture for a few seconds while breathing regularly.

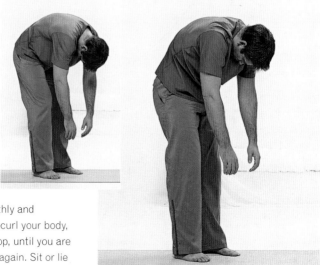

4 Slowly, smoothly and attentively uncurl your body, from bottom to top, until you are standing upright again. Sit or lie down and rest.

progressive relaxation

Reduces anxiety levels and high blood pressure
Improves concentration and sleep patterns
Increases ability to cope with pain and to manage stress

1 Lie on your back on a mat. Separate your feet slightly and move your arms from your sides. Keep your arms straight but relaxed, and the palms of your hands upturned. Close your eyes. Unclench your teeth so that you relax your jaw, but keep your lips lightly closed. Breathe regularly through your nose.

2 Focus your attention on your feet. Pull your toes towards you and push your heels away from you. Hold this ankle position briefly but keep breathing regularly. Now relax your ankles and feet. Next shift your attention to your knees. Stiffen your legs to 'lock' your knee joints. Briefly hold the tension then relax your knees and legs.

3 Tighten your buttock muscles. Hold the tightness for a few seconds but keep breathing regularly. Release the tightness and then relax your hips.

Progressive relaxation is the gradual and conscious letting go of built-up tension in the body's muscles.

4 Exhale and press the small of your back (at waist level) towards or against the mat. Hold the pressure as long as your exhalation lasts. Release the pressure as you inhale. Continue to breathe regularly.

5 Inhale and squeeze your shoulder blades together. Hold the squeeze as long as your inhalation lasts. Release the squeeze as you exhale. Continue to breathe regularly.

6 On an exhalation, tighten your abdominal muscles. Hold the tightness while the exhalation lasts. Inhale and then relax. Continue breathing regularly.

7 Take a slow, smooth, deep inhalation, imagining that you are filling the top, middle and bottom of your lungs. Be aware of your chest expanding and your abdomen rising. Exhale slowly, smoothly and steadily, imagining that you are emptying your lungs by degrees. Be conscious of your chest and abdomen relaxing. Resume regular breathing.

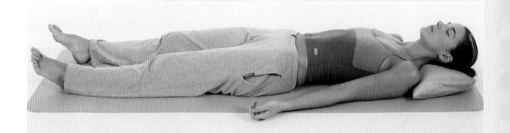

8 Tighten your hands into fists, straighten your arms and raise them off the mat. Hold the stiffness briefly but keep breathing regularly. Then let your arms and hands fall to the mat, free of stiffness. Relax both your elbow joints and your wrists.

9 Keep your arms relaxed but shrug your shoulders, as if to touch your ears with them. Briefly hold the shrug then relax your shoulders.

10 Gently roll your head from side to side a few times. Reposition your head and check that you are still breathing in a regular pattern.

11 Exhaling, open your eyes and mouth widely; stick out your tongue; tense all your facial muscles, just like a menacing lion. Inhale, close your mouth and eyes and then relax your facial muscles again.

12 Spend a few moments visualizing all of the tension draining from your face and eyes.

13 Lie relaxed for as many minutes as you can spare. Surrender your body to the surface that supports it. Each time you exhale, let your body sink more deeply. Each time you inhale, imagine you are filling your system with peace and tranquillity.

14 Before getting up, rotate your ankles a few times; gently roll your head from side to side; leisurely stretch your limbs. Get up slowly and safely.

TIPS

- If you are unwell or are recovering from an illness or from surgery, you may practise Progressive Relaxation in bed or in an easy chair. Use whatever props you need to support your body, particularly your neck and lower back, so that you are absolutely comfortable.

- Keep a jumper or a blanket and a pair of warm socks nearby. Use them if necessary to prevent you from becoming cold as your body cools down during relaxation.

- You may want to use some imagery in step 13 or simply do some visualization. You may, for example, visualize yourself lying on a warm, sandy beach in summer, with a gentle breeze caressing your face, hair and body, as you revel in pleasant memories.

- Practise Progressive Relaxation whenever you feel tired, anxious or otherwise stressed. When you have become well versed in the technique, you may dispense with alternately tensing and relaxing muscle groups and simply give mental suggestion to the various parts to let go of tension and relax. For example, you may focus attention on your abdomen and mentally say to it: 'Abdomen, let go of your tightness. Relax.'

- Practise Progressive Relaxation anywhere it is convenient for you to do so. Ideally, the technique is best done in a quiet place for 10 to 20 minutes where you won't be interrupted.

- You may find it helpful to read the instructions for this exercise into a tape-recorder, or ask a friend to do so. Speak slowly and soothingly.

rhythmic diaphragmatic breathing

Increases exercise tolerance
Helps when coping with pain, anxiety and other forms of stress
Improves both the ability to relax and quality of sleep at night

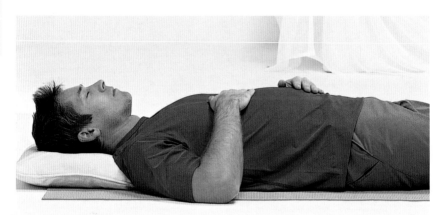

1 Lie at full length on your back, with a pillow, cushion or folded towel under your head. Close your eyes or keep them open. Relax your jaw and breathe regularly. Rest one hand lightly on your abdomen, just beneath your breastbone. Rest the fingers of your other hand on your chest, just below the nipple. Keeping your abdomen as relaxed as possible, inhale through your nose slowly, smoothly and as fully as you can without strain. As you do so, the hand on the abdomen should rise as the abdomen moves upwards. There should be little or no movement of the fingers resting on the chest.

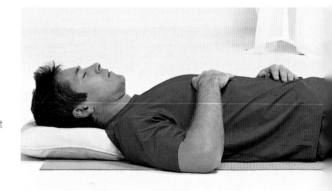

2 Exhale through your nose slowly, smoothly and as completely as you can without using any force. As you do so, the hand on the abdomen should move downwards as the abdomen contracts (tightens). Repeat the exercise several times in smooth succession. Relax your arms and hands. Breathe regularly.

TIPS

- It may help you to pick up this breathing technique if you exhale through pursed lips, as if cooling a hot drink or whistling. If you start to feel lightheaded, though, resume normal breathing immediately. (And if you are standing, sit down.)

- If in doubt whether your abdomen should rise or fall on inhalation, think of a balloon: as you put air into it, it becomes larger; when you let the air out, it becomes flat. To help you remember, try saying this phrase over and over to yourself: 'Air in, abdomen fat; air out, abdomen flat.'

- When first learning this breathing technique, place a light object – a small pillow, a rubber duck or boat or a paper plane – on your abdomen, to provide visual feedback. It should rise on inhalation and fall on exhalation.

- When you have mastered rhythmic diaphragmatic breathing lying down, try it sitting, standing or in a semi-reclining position. Coordinate it with activities such as vacuum-cleaning, raking leaves or walking up and down stairs.

child's pose

Eases pressure on spinal discs
Keeps the spine flexible
Improves circulation and elimination of wastes
Promotes overall relaxation

Kneel with your legs together and your body upright but relaxed and your feet pointing backwards. Slowly lower your body to sit on your heels. Breathe regularly. Slowly bend forwards and rest your forehead on the mat or turn your head to the side. Relax your arms with palms up at your sides. Stay like this as long as you are comfortable. Breathe regularly: with each outgoing breath, visualize sending away tiredness, anxiety and other difficult feelings. Slowly resume a sitting position. Stretch out and rest.

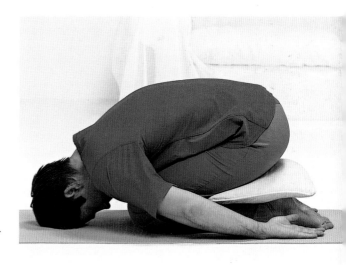

VARIATION

You may find it more comfortable to rest your forehead on a cushion or pillow. Place a folded towel or pillow between your bottom and feet, if you wish.

main exercises

The following exercises are designed to be practised in the programmes (see pages 108 to 121). If you are doing the exercises for the first time, or have not been exercising regularly or are recovering from an injury or illness, please follow the **BEGINNER**'s instructions; omit any exercise where **BEGINNER** is not mentioned. After a few weeks of regular practice, you may progress to the **INTERMEDIATE** level; the **ADVANCED** category is for those who are fit and strong.

chest expansion

Reduces tension build-up in the shoulders and upper back
Helps to improve posture
Facilitates deep breathing
Helps prevent osteoporosis

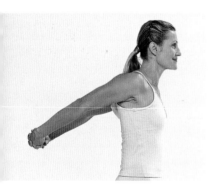

Stand tall with your feet comfortably apart and your weight equally distributed between them. Relax your jaw and breathe regularly through your nose. Inhale and swing your arms behind you; interlace the fingers of one hand with those of the other. Exhale. Inhale and raise the linked hands as high as you comfortably can. Maintain good posture. Hold the raised-arms position for a few seconds while breathing slowly and smoothly. Exhale and lower your arms; relax them at your sides. Rest.

BEGINNER
2 times; hold 6 seconds

INTERMEDIATE
2 times; hold 8 seconds

ADVANCED
2 times; hold 10 seconds

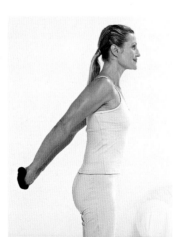

VARIATION
You may practise Chest Expansion with a 1–1.5 kg (2–3 lb) weight in each hand by squeezing your shoulder blades together instead of interlacing your fingers.

posture clasp

Keeps the shoulder joints moving freely
Prevents stiffness and promotes good posture
Facilitates deep breathing

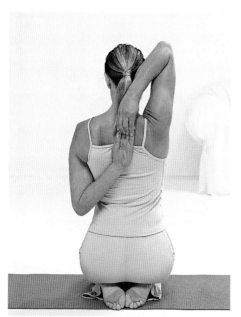
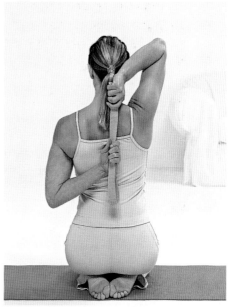

Sit or stand tall. Relax your jaw and breathe regularly through your nose throughout the exercise. Reach over your right shoulder with your right hand. Point your elbow straight upwards and keep your arm close to your ear. With your left hand, reach behind you from below and interlock your fingers with those of your right hand. Maintain good posture. Hold this position for a few seconds while breathing regularly. Relax your arms and hands. Repeat the exercise, changing hands.

VARIATION

If you are unable to link your hands together, use a scarf, belt or other aid as an extension to your arms. Pull upwards on one end and downwards on the other.

BEGINNER
2 times; hold 6 seconds

INTERMEDIATE
3 times; hold 8 seconds

ADVANCED
3 times; hold 10 seconds

half moon

Promotes flexibility of the spine
Provides lateral (sideways) bending and stretching to strengthen abdominal muscles
Facilitates deep breathing

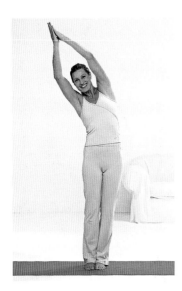

Stand tall, with your feet together and body weight distributed evenly. Relax your jaw and breathe regularly through your nose. Inhale, raise your arms to the side and then bring them overhead with your palms together if you can. Exhale and bend your upper body slowly and smoothly to one side, to form a graceful arc, like a half moon. Check the bend is sideways not forward. Hold this posture for a few seconds but keep breathing regularly. Inhale and come upright. Relax your arms. Rest briefly. Repeat the exercise on the other side. Rest.

BEGINNER 2 times; hold 6 seconds

INTERMEDIATE 2 times; hold 8 seconds

ADVANCED 2 times; hold 10 seconds

sideways stretch

Encourages good posture while sitting
Keeps the spine flexible
Strengthens abdominal muscles

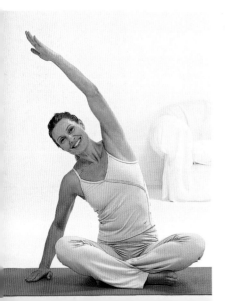

Sit comfortably with your legs folded inwards. Relax the jaw and breathe regularly through your nose. Rest one palm on the mat beside your hip, with fingers pointing forwards. Exhale, raise your free arm overhead and slowly and smoothly bend your upper body sideways towards the hand on the mat. Keep your upper arm aligned with your ear. Hold this posture for a few seconds while breathing regularly. Inhale and come upright. Relax your arm. Rest briefly. Repeat the exercise on the other side. Rest.

BEGINNER 2 times; hold 6 seconds

INTERMEDIATE 2 times; hold 8 seconds

ADVANCED 2 times; hold 10 seconds

Pilates spine twist

Gives gentle torsion (twisting) to the spine
Stretches and strengthens lower back muscles
Strengthens abdominal muscles
Helps build bone mass and prevent osteoporosis

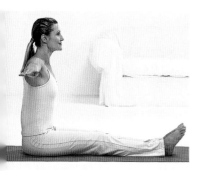

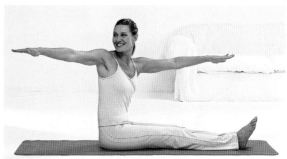

1 Sit tall, with the crown of your head uppermost and your legs stretched out in front. Relax your jaw and breathe regularly through your nose. Inhale and stretch your arms out sideways in line with your shoulders.

2 Exhaling, slowly and smoothly swivel your body to the right, from the waist up, keeping your hips facing forwards. Look to the right. Hold this posture for a few seconds while breathing regularly. Inhale and swivel your body back to the centre. Repeat the exercise on the other side.

VARIATION

If you hold a 1–1.5 kg (2–3 lb) weight in each hand, the exercise can help in protecting against bone loss through osteoporosis.

BEGINNER
2 times; hold 6 seconds

INTERMEDIATE
3 times; hold 8 seconds

ADVANCED
3 times; hold 10 seconds

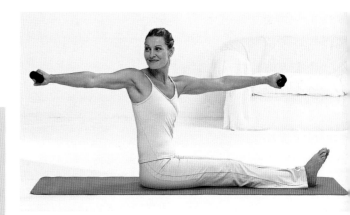

yoga spinal twist

Gives maximum torsion to the spine and so promotes range of motion

Gently massages the lower back muscles

Strengthens the abdominal muscles

1 Sit tall with your legs stretched out in front. Relax your jaw and breathe regularly through your nose.

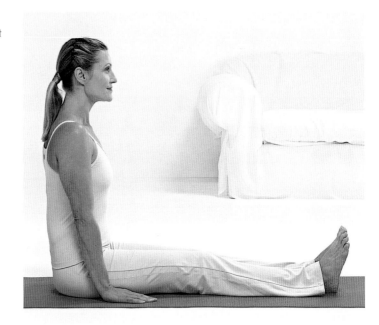

2 Bend your left leg and place your left foot beside your outer right knee. Exhaling, slowly and smoothly rotate your upper body to the left. Rest one or both hands on the mat at your left side. Look to the left. Hold this posture for a few seconds while breathing regularly.

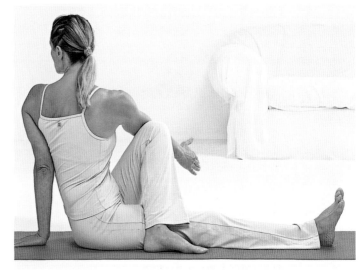

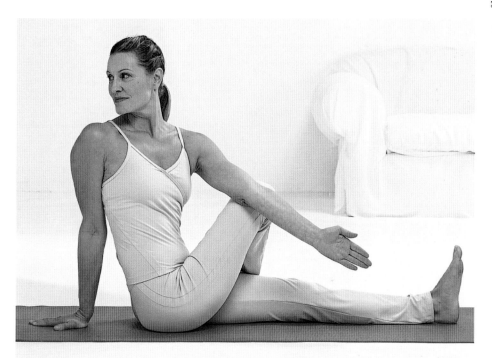

3 Inhale and slowly return to your starting position. Rest. Breathe regularly. Repeat the exercise, this time twisting to the other side.

BEGINNER
Hold 6 seconds

INTERMEDIATE
Hold 8 seconds

ADVANCED
Hold 10 or more seconds

single-leg raise

Strengthens the abdominal muscles
Gently stretches the hamstrings to prevent shortening
Exercises the back muscles

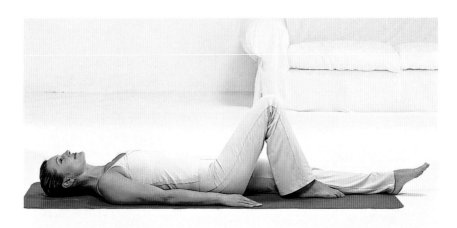

1 Lie flat on your back. Keep one leg stretched out in front and the other bent with the sole of the foot on the mat. Relax your arms at your sides. Breathe regularly.

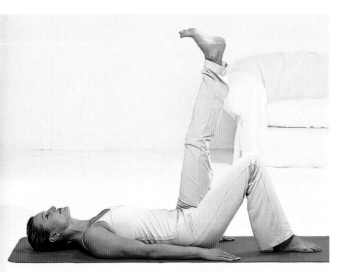

2 Press the small of your back to the mat. Exhale and raise the straight leg, slowly and with control, until your lower abdomen tightens. Hold the raised-leg posture as long as you comfortably can while breathing regularly. Slowly and with control, lower the leg to the mat while inhaling. Rest briefly. Repeat these steps with the same leg, then do it with the other leg the same number of times. Rest afterwards.

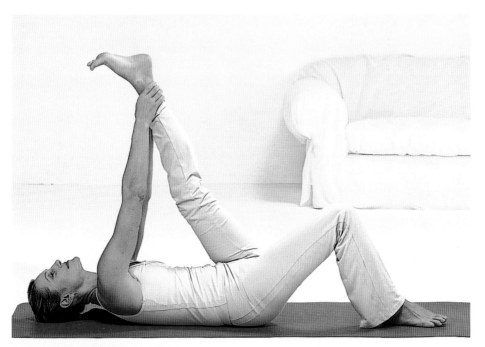

VARIATION
Pull the toes of your raised leg
towards you and push away with
the heel for a therapeutic stretch
to the hamstring muscles down
the back of your thigh.

BEGINNER
3 times; hold 6 seconds

INTERMEDIATE
5 times; hold 8 seconds

ADVANCED
6 times; hold 10 seconds

little abdominal curl

Strengthens back muscles
Keeps the spine flexible
Strengthens the abdominal muscles
Strengthens the inner thigh muscles when
using a ball

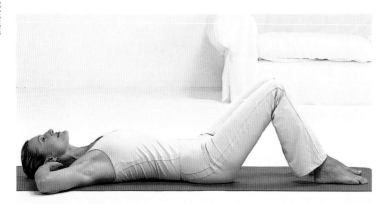

1 Lie on your back with your hands placed under your head. (You may also rest your head on a thin pillow.) To ensure the correct head position, imagine holding a small orange or a tennis ball securely between your jaw and your throat. Bend your legs and rest the soles of your feet flat on the mat, a comfortable distance from your bottom.

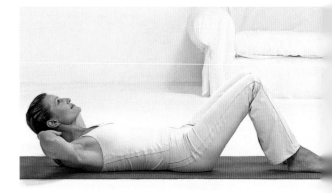

2 Exhale and carefully raise your head, still supported by your hands, to gaze at your thighs. Hold this position for a few seconds while breathing regularly. Inhale and carefully lower your head to resume your starting position. Relax your arms and legs. Rest.

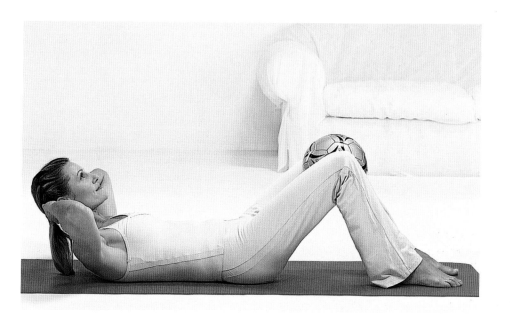

VARIATION (WITH BALL)

Start as in step 1 left, but place an
exercise ball between your knees
and make sure it is secure as you
proceed to step 2.

BEGINNER
3 times; hold 6 seconds

INTERMEDIATE
4 times; hold 8 seconds

ADVANCED
5 times; hold 10 seconds

roll up

Strengthens the rectus abdominis muscles, which run up and down the front of the abdomen
Strengthens the back muscles
Keeps the spine flexible

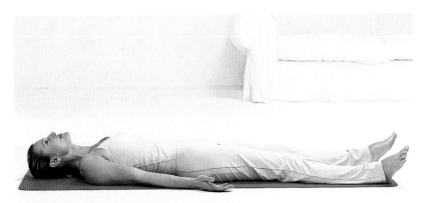

1 Lie on your back, with your legs stretched out in front and slightly separated. Relax your jaw and breathe regularly.

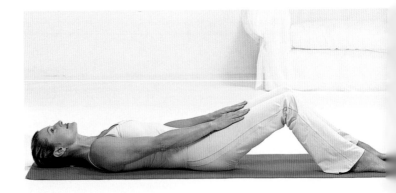

2 Bend your knees and slide your feet towards your bottom until the soles are flat on the mat. Maintain this distance between feet and bottom as you do the Roll Up. Rest your palms on the front of your thighs.

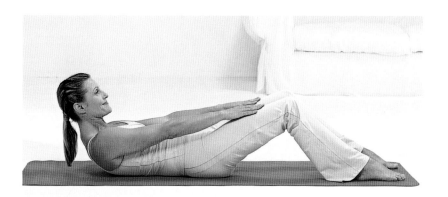

3 Exhaling, slowly raise your head. Keep your gaze on your hands while sliding them towards your knees.

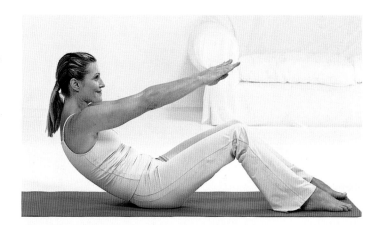

4 When you feel the most tension tolerable in your abdomen, stop. Hold the posture as long as you are absolutely comfortable (you may raise your hands). Breathe regularly. Inhale and slowly curl your spine back on to the mat. Stretch your legs, relax your arms at your sides and rest.

INTERMEDIATE
2 times; hold 8 seconds
or as tolerated

ADVANCED
2 times; hold 10 seconds
or as tolerated

diagonal curl up

Strengthens the transverse and oblique abdominal muscles
Strengthens back muscles
Keeps the spine flexible
Strengthens inner thigh muscles when using a ball

1 Lie on your back, with your knees bent and the soles of your feet flat on the mat. Relax your arms at your sides. Breathe regularly.

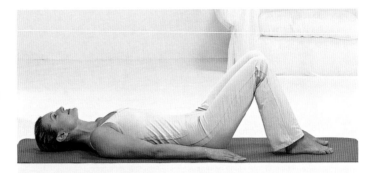

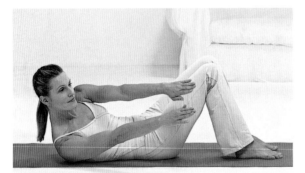

2 Exhaling, slowly curl your upper body forwards, reaching with both hands towards the outside of your right knee. Hold this posture for several seconds but keep breathing regularly. Slowly uncurl your body on to the mat, stretch out your legs and relax your arms at your sides. Rest briefly. Repeat on the other side. Rest.

VARIATION

Start as in step 1 above, but also securely position an exercise ball between your bent knees. Proceed to step 2 above.

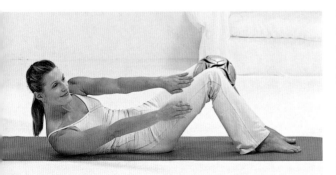

INTERMEDIATE
2 times; hold 8 seconds

ADVANCED
2 times; hold 10 seconds

pelvic tilt

Increases flexibility of the spine
Strengthens the abdominal and lower back muscles
Relieves stiffness and minor backaches

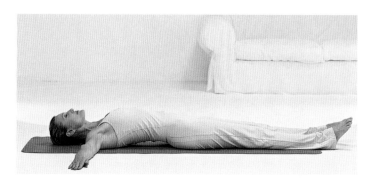

1 Lie on your back with your legs stretched out in front. Breathe regularly.

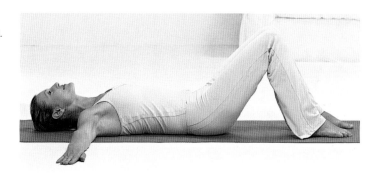

2 Bend your legs and rest the soles of your feet comfortably flat on the mat. (You can also do the Pelvic Tilt while sitting or standing, or in an all-fours position as in the Cat Stretch on page 104.) On exhalation, slowly press the small of your back downwards, to decrease the spinal arch. You will then feel your abdomen tighten and your pelvis tilt slightly upwards. Hold the pressure and pelvic tilt for a few seconds while breathing regularly. Inhale and relax. Stretch out your legs and rest. Breathe regularly.

BEGINNER
3 times; hold 6 seconds

INTERMEDIATE
4 times; hold 8 seconds

ADVANCED
5 times; hold 10 seconds

teaser (modified)

Strengthens abdominal muscles to provide efficient support for the back
Develops concentration, coordination and balance

1 Sit tall, with your legs bent and the soles of your feet flat on the mat in front of you. Breathe regularly through your nose.

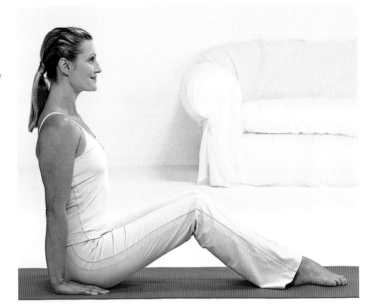

2 Tilt backwards to balance on your bottom; bring your legs closer to your body and lift your feet off the mat (use your hands for balance, if necessary). Stretch out your arms so they are parallel to the mat. Straighten your legs, slowly and with control.

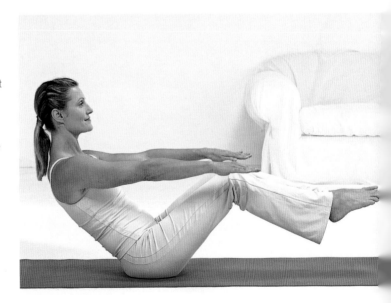

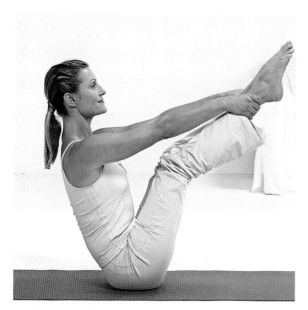

3 Adjust your degree of tilt to help you maintain balance (hold your ankles if this helps). Keep your gaze on your legs. Hold this posture for a few seconds, focusing attention on your regular breathing to help you stay steady. Slowly and carefully resume your starting position: bring your knees to your chest and rest your hands on the mat to help. Sit or lie down and have a rest.

VARIATION
Try stretching your arms upwards, parallel to your raised legs. Keep your gaze on your arms.

INTERMEDIATE
Hold 8 seconds

ADVANCED
Hold 10 seconds

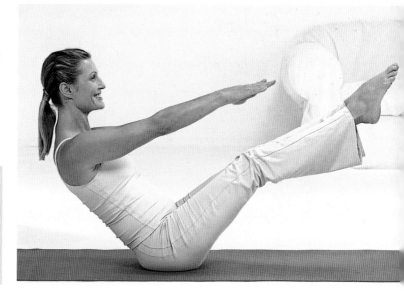

the bridge

Strengthens the back muscles
Increases the flexibility of the spine
Stretches and strengthens the abdominal and thigh muscles

1 Lie on your back with your legs stretched in front and your arms relaxed at your sides. Turn your palms downwards. Breathe regularly. Bend your legs and rest the soles of your feet flat on the mat, at a comfortable distance from your bottom.

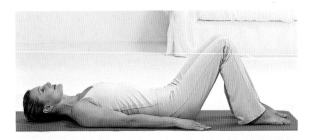

2 Inhaling, raise first your hips then slowly and smoothly the rest of your back, until your torso is fully raised and straight. Hold the posture for several seconds while breathing regularly. Slowly and smoothly lower your torso from top to bottom, one vertebra at a time, until it is flat on the mat once more. Synchronize your movement with regular breathing. Stretch out your legs. Relax your hands. Rest.

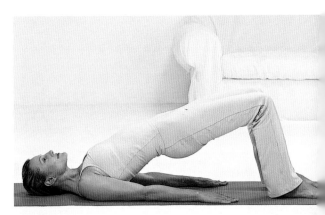

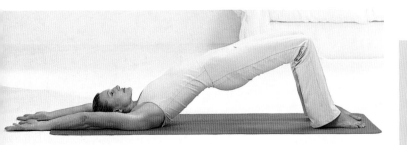

VARIATION
This variation gives the whole body a therapeutic stretch. Once your body is fully raised, stretch your arms overhead. Point your knees forwards and your fingers backwards to intensify the stretch to the muscles at the front of your body.

BEGINNER
2 times; hold 6 seconds

INTERMEDIATE
3 times; hold 10 seconds

ADVANCED
4 times; hold 10 or more seconds

double-leg stretch

Strengthens muscles of the abdomen, neck, shoulders and back

Relieves back fatigue, back strain and backache

Lie on your back, with your legs stretched out in front and your arms at your sides. (Rest your head on a small pillow, if necessary.) Breathe regularly. Bring first one bent knee, then the other, towards your chest, each time on an exhalation, and hold them securely in place with your hands or arms. Hold this position for several seconds while breathing regularly. Synchronizing your movement with regular breathing, release your hold on your legs and stretch them out again, one at a time. Relax your arms and hands.

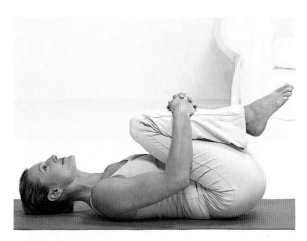

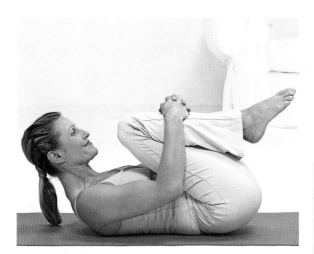

VARIATION (INTERMEDIATE AND ADVANCED)
Once you are holding your knees, carefully lift your head, bringing it towards your knees. Make sure you lower your head carefully before releasing your legs.

BEGINNER
Hold 6 to 10
seconds or longer

INTERMEDIATE
Variation; hold 8
or more seconds

ADVANCED
Variation; hold 10
or more seconds

swan dive

Keeps the spine flexible
Strengthens the back muscles
Stretches and strengthens the muscles at the front of the torso

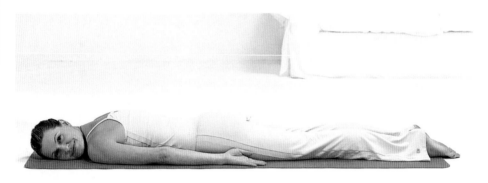

1 Lie on your front, with your head turned to the side. Relax your arms at your sides. Breathe regularly.

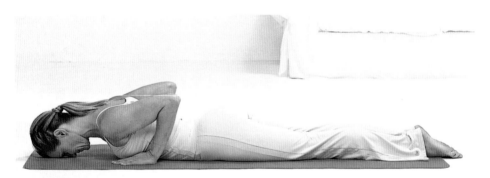

2 Turn your head to the front. Rest your forehead on the mat. Place your palms on the mat so that they are directly beneath your shoulders and keep your arms close to your sides.

BEGINNER
2 times; hold 6 seconds

INTERMEDIATE
2 times; hold 8 seconds

ADVANCED
2 times; hold 10 or more seconds

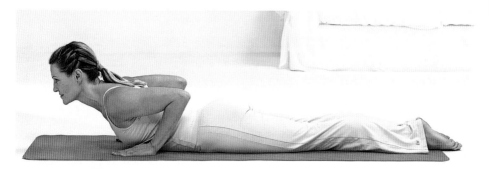

3 Inhaling, slowly and carefully lift your head and gently arch your back in one smooth movement. Breathe regularly and continue this controlled arching of your back as far as you can manage without straining. Hold this posture for several seconds while breathing regularly. Slowly and smoothly come out of the posture, from bottom to top, one vertebra at a time. Rest in your starting position.

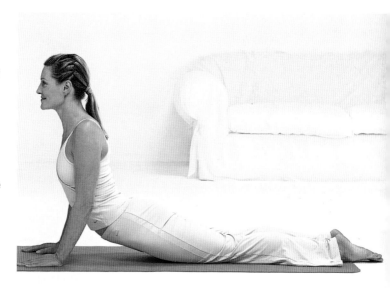

VARIATION
Following steps 2 and 3 left and above, slowly and smoothly arch your back as far as your shoulders, on an inhalation.

rocking

Keeps the spine flexible
Strengthens the back muscles
Strengthens the abdominal muscles
Strengthens the legs

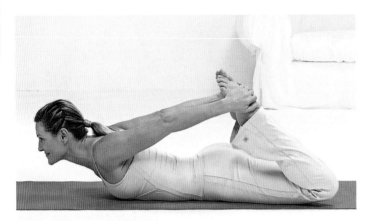

1 Lie face downwards, with your legs comfortably separated and your arms at your sides. Breathe regularly. Bend your knees and bring your feet in towards your bottom. Carefully tilt your head back; reach for your feet, one at a time, and grasp your ankles. Keep breathing regularly.

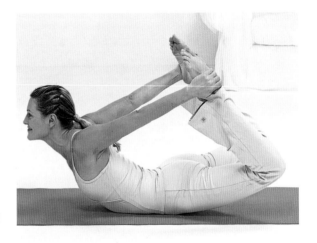

2 Exhaling, push your feet upwards and away from you. This action will raise your legs and arch your body. Hold this posture for several seconds. As you inhale and exhale while doing so, your body will move backwards and forwards like a rocking-horse. Carefully return to your starting position. Relax your arms and hands. Rest.

ADVANCED
Hold 5 to 10 seconds

prone leg raise

Strengthens the back and the legs
Stretches and strengthens the abdominal muscles

Lie on your front, with your legs close together and your chin on the mat. Breathe regularly. Straighten your arms and position them at your sides. Make your hands into fists. Raise one leg as high as you comfortably can while exhaling. Keep your chin, arms, hands and body pressed to the mat. Hold the raised-leg posture for several seconds while breathing regularly. Lower your leg to the mat, slowly and with control. Synchronize the movement with regular breathing. Rest briefly. Repeat with the other leg.

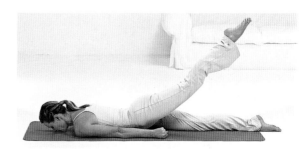

BEGINNER 3 times; hold 6 seconds

INTERMEDIATE 3 times; hold 8 seconds

ADVANCED 3 times; hold 10 seconds

swimming

Strengthens the muscles of the back, legs and arms
Stretches and strengthens the abdominal and other muscles at the front of the body

Lie on your front. Rest your chin on the mat. Stretch your legs out and put your arms in front. Breathe regularly. Inhale and lift your right arm and left leg at the same time. Slightly lift your head but do not arch your neck. Look straight ahead. Hold this position for a few seconds while breathing regularly. Exhaling, lower your arm and leg, then inhale and lift your left arm and right leg. Hold this position for a few seconds while breathing regularly. Repeat the exercise several times in smooth succession, visualizing yourself swimming in the ocean. Return to

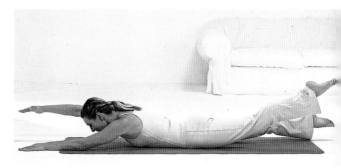

your starting position. Turn your head to the side and relax your arms and legs. Rest. (A good position in which to rest is the Child's Pose, on page 79.)

ADVANCED
3 to 5 times; hold
3 to 5 seconds

dog stretch

Helps maintain the elasticity of the hamstring muscles
Relaxes tired legs and also the rest of the body

1 Start in an all-fours position on your hands and knees, with your arms sloping slightly forwards. Breathe regularly.

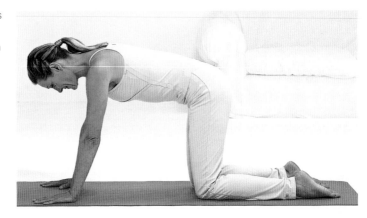

2 Tuck in your toes so that they point forwards. Rock backwards slightly. Raise your knees and straighten your legs. Straighten your arms. Now you are in a hips-high, head-low posture. Aim your heels towards the mat without straining the muscles at the back of your legs. Stay in this posture for several seconds while breathing regularly. Gently rock forwards and slowly return to your starting position. Sit on your heels, with your toes pointing backwards, and rest. (Or rest in any other comfortable position.)

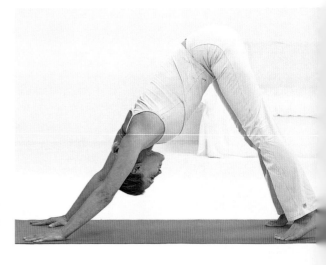

BEGINNER Hold 6 seconds

INTERMEDIATE Hold 8 seconds

ADVANCED Hold 10 seconds

single-leg kicks

Stretches and strengthens the leg muscles, particularly those of the thighs

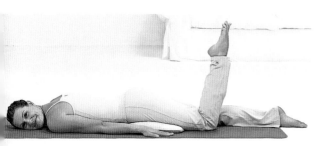

Lie on your front, with your face turned to the side. Keep your legs together and your arms relaxed at your sides. (A thin cushion or folded towel under your hips will prevent accentuation of the spinal arch at the small of your back.) Breathe regularly. Slowly bend one leg, bringing the heel towards your bottom. Enjoy the stretch in the thigh muscles. Synchronize the leg movement with regular breathing. Hold the bent-leg position for a few seconds, breathing regularly. Rest the bent leg on the mat. Repeat with the other leg.

BEGINNER 3 times; hold 6 seconds

INTERMEDIATE 4 times; hold 8 seconds

ADVANCED 5 times; hold 10 seconds

quadriceps stretch, standing

Strengthens the leg muscles, particularly those of the thighs
Promotes concentration and develops nerve/muscle coordination (variation)

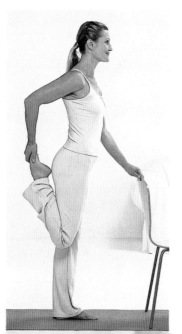

Stand tall, near a chair or other stable prop, with your feet a little apart and your weight evenly distributed. Breathe regularly. Shift your weight on to your left foot. Bend your right leg and point your foot backwards. Grasp the foot with your right hand and bring it as close to your buttock as is comfortable. If necessary, hold the prop with your free hand for balance. Hold the posture for several seconds while breathing regularly. Slowly resume your starting position. Rest briefly. Repeat, standing on your right foot this time.

BEGINNER
2 times; hold 6 seconds

INTERMEDIATE
2 times; hold 8 seconds

ADVANCED
2 times; hold 10 seconds

cat stretch

Keeps the spine flexible
Strengthens back and abdominal muscles
Relieves stiffness and minor backaches

1 Start in an all-fours position on your hands and knees and with your back level. Breathe regularly.

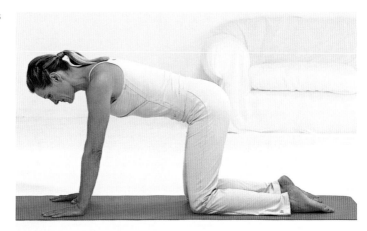

2 On an exhalation, lower your head, tuck your bottom down and arch your back and shoulders, slowly and smoothly, focusing your attention mostly on the pelvic movement rather than your shoulders. Imagine yourself as a cat with its back rounded. This is the Pelvic Tilt (see page 93) in an all-fours position. Hold the stretch for a few seconds and breathe regularly. Resume the starting position, synchronizing your movement with regular breathing. Sit on your heels or in any comfortable position and rest.

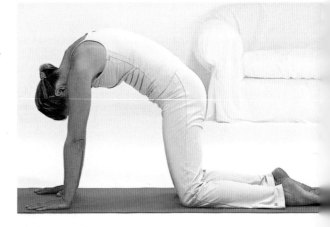

BEGINNER 3 times; hold 6 seconds

INTERMEDIATE 4 times; hold 8 seconds

ADVANCED 4 times; hold 10 seconds

squatting

Eases pressure on spinal discs
Relaxes the muscles and ligaments of the back
Strengthens the legs

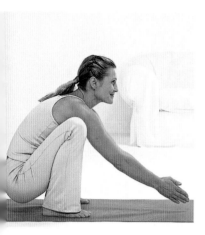

Stand with your feet comfortably apart and your weight evenly distributed. Breathe regularly through your nose. Exhaling, slowly bend your knees as if to sit, until your bottom is close to your heels. Arrange your arms comfortably. Hold this posture for a few seconds, breathing regularly, or alternate it with returning to the start position several times in smooth succession. Inhale and then slowly return to your starting position.

BEGINNER
3 times; hold 6 seconds or more

INTERMEDIATE
4 times; hold 8 seconds or more

ADVANCED
5 times; hold 10 seconds or more

wall squat

Strengthens the legs
Encourages good posture in standing
Strengthens the abdominal and back muscles
Builds bone and helps prevent osteoporosis

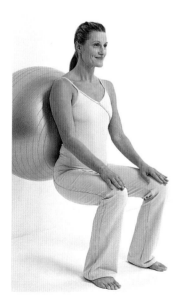

Stand tall with your back to a wall. Put an exercise ball securely between your waist and the wall. Maintain good posture. Relax your jaw and breathe regularly through your nose. Exhaling, bend your knees as if preparing to sit down, until your thighs are parallel to the mat. Keep your abdominal muscles tight and your back parallel to the wall. Hold for a few seconds, breathing regularly. Inhale and slowly reverse your movement to return to your starting position. (As you squat, the ball will move to your mid- and upper-back and roll down again as you resume your starting position.) Repeat then rest.

INTERMEDIATE
3 to 5 times; hold 5 seconds

ADVANCED
8 times; hold 5 to 10 seconds

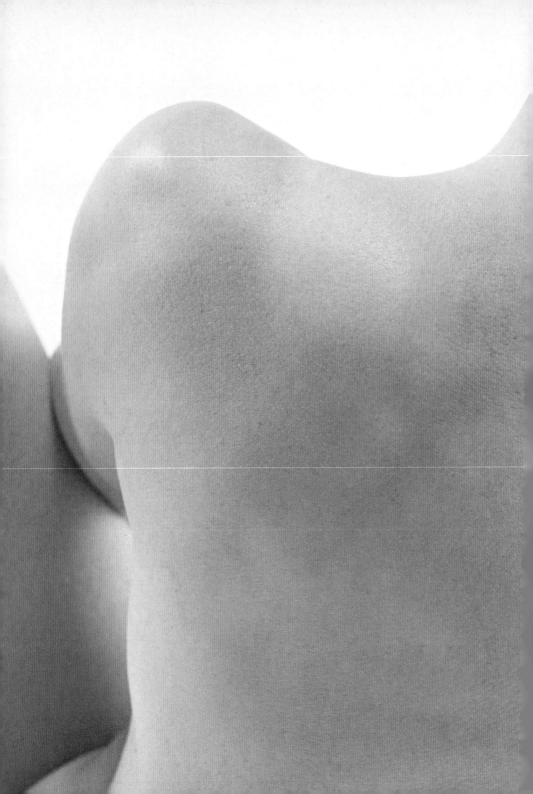

back programmes

Depending on your fitness level and your degree of discomfort due to back pain, try spending about two weeks on each of the following routines before progressing to the next. Try to practise the suggested programme every day if you can, but in any case at least every other day. If you cannot spare the required 15 to 20 minutes per session, you can opt for the shortened versions (see pages 114–119) and incorporate whatever other exercise you can into your daily activities. The exercises have been arranged to make the transition from one to the next as smooth and logical as possible. If this order doesn't feel quite right for you, then please choose the sequence that suits you best. It is important that you are comfortable and that you enjoy doing them.

beginner

warm-ups

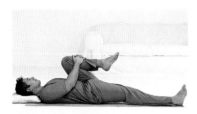

Single-Knee Hug, p. 69

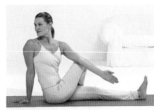

Yoga Spinal Twist, p. 84–85

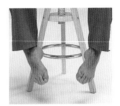

Foot Circles, p. 67

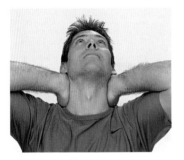

Neck Stretch, p. 65

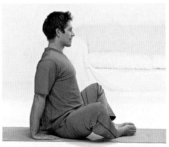

Butterfly (variation), p. 68

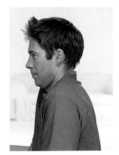

Shoulder Circle, p. 66 or Arm Circle with weights, p. 67

main exercises

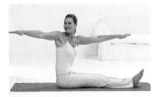

Pilates Spine Twist, p. 83

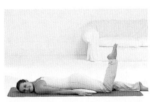

Single-Leg Kicks, p. 103

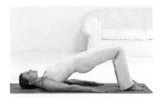

The Bridge, p. 96

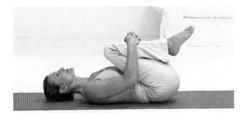

Double-Leg Stretch, p. 97

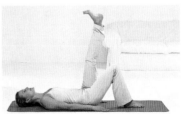

Single-Leg Raise, p. 86

main exercises continued

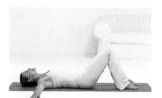

Pelvic Tilt, p. 93

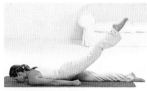

Prone Leg Raise, p. 101

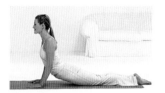

Swan Dive (variation), p. 98–99

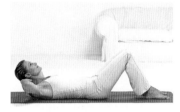

Little Abdominal Curl (with or without ball), p. 88

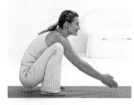

Squatting, p. 105

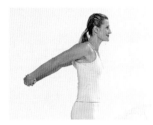

Chest Expansion (with or without weights), p. 80

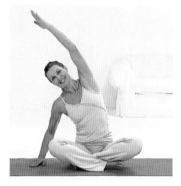

Half Moon or Sideways Stretch, p. 82

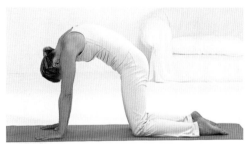

Cat Stretch, p. 104

cool down

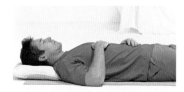

Progressive Relaxation, p. 76–77, or Rhythmic Diaphragmatic Breathing, p. 78

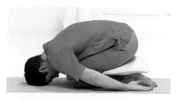

or in Child's Pose, p. 79

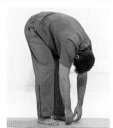

or Roll Down, p. 74–75

intermediate

warm-ups

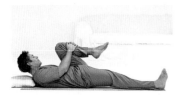

Single-Knee Hug (variation), p. 69

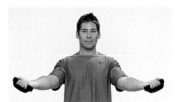

Shoulder Circle, p. 66 or Arm Circle with weights, p. 67

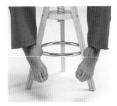

Foot Circles, p. 67

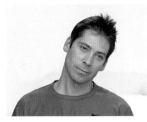

Neck Stretch, p. 65, including Chin Glide (turtle), p. 64

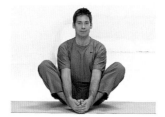

Butterfly, p. 68

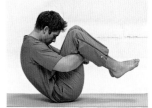

Rolling Like a Ball, p. 72

main exercises

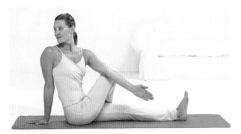

Yoga Spinal Twist, p. 84–85

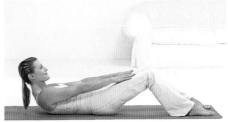

Roll Up, p. 90–91

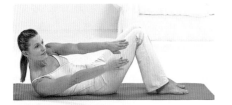

Diagonal Curl Up (with or without ball), p. 92

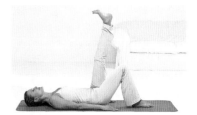

Single-Leg Raise, p. 86

main exercises continued

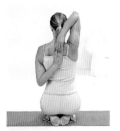

Posture Clasp, p. 81

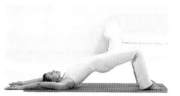

The Bridge (variation), p. 96

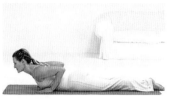

Swan Dive, p. 98–99

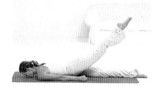

Prone Leg Raise, p. 101

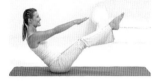

Teaser (modified), p. 94–95

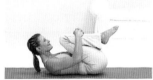

Double-Leg Stretch (variation), p. 97

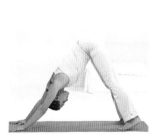

Dog Stretch, p. 102

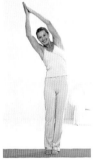

Half Moon, p. 82

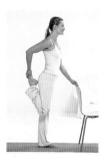

Quadriceps Stretch, standing, p. 103

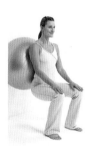

Wall Squat, p. 105

cool down

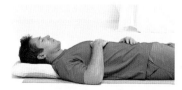

Progressive Relaxation, p. 76–77, or
Rhythmic Diaphragmatic Breathing, p. 78

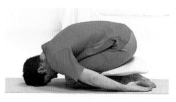

or in Child's Pose, p. 79

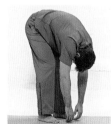

or Roll Down, p. 74–75

advanced

warm-ups

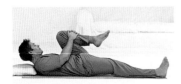

Single-Knee Hug (variation), p. 69

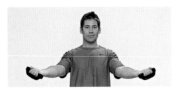

Shoulder Circle or Arm Circle with weights, p. 66–67

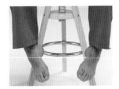

Foot Circle, p. 67

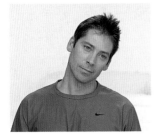

Neck Stretch, p. 65, including Chin Glide (turtle), p. 64

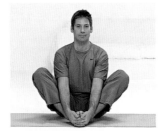

Butterfly, p. 68

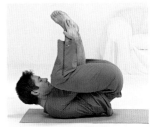

Seal, p. 73

main exercises

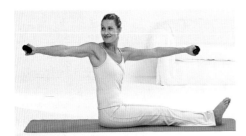

Pilates Spine Twist (variation), p. 83

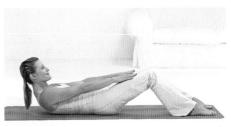

Roll Up, p. 90–91

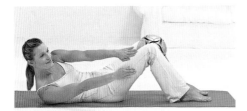

Pelvic Tilt, p. 93

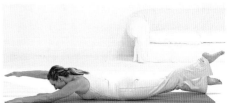

Squatting, p. 105

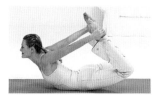

Rocking, p. 100

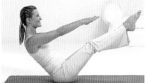

Teaser (modified), p. 94–95

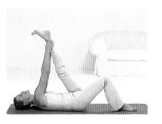

Single-Leg Raise (variation), p. 86

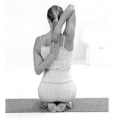

Posture Clasp, p. 81

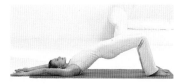

The Bridge (variation), p. 96

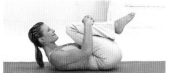

Double-Leg Stretch (variation), p. 97

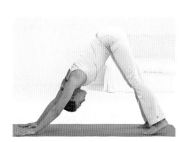

Dog Stretch, p. 102

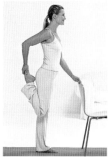

Quadriceps Stretch, standing
(with or without prop), p. 103

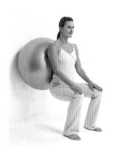

Wall Squat, p. 105

cool down

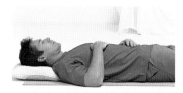

Progressive Relaxation, p. 76–77, or
Rhythmic Diaphragmatic Breathing, p. 78

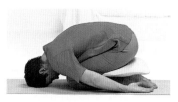

or in Child's Pose, p. 79

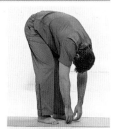

or Roll Down, p. 74–75

shortened programmes – beginner

warm-ups

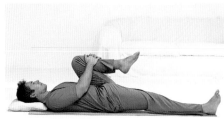

Single-Knee Hug, p 69

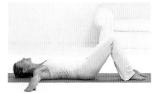

Lying Twist (variation), p. 70

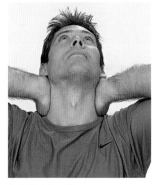

Neck Stretch, p. 65

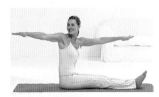

Butterfly (variation), p. 68

main exercises

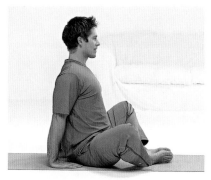

Pilates Spinal Twist, p. 83

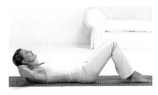

Little Abdominal Curl (with or without ball), p. 88

Pelvic Tilt, p. 93

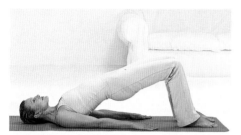

The Bridge, p. 96

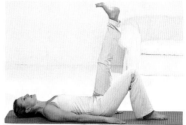

Single-Leg Raise, p. 86

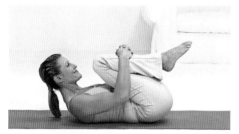

Double-Leg Stretch, p. 97

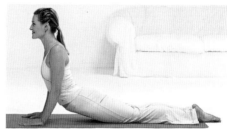

Swan Dive (variation), p. 98–99

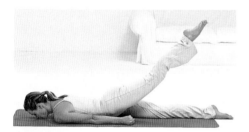

Prone Leg Raise, p. 101

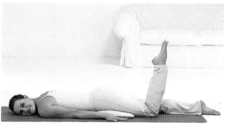

Single-Leg Kicks, p. 103

cool down

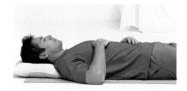

Progressive Relaxation, p. 76–77, or
Rhythmic Diaphragmatic Breathing, p. 78

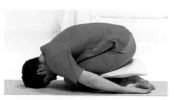

or in Child's Pose, p. 79

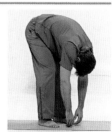

or Roll Down, p. 74–75

shortened programmes – intermediate

warm-ups

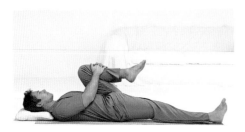

Single-Knee Hug, p. 69

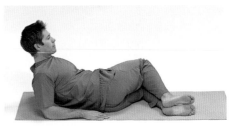

Lying Twist (variation), p. 70

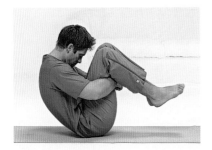

Rolling Like a Ball, p. 72

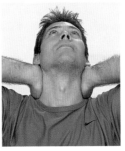

Neck Stretch, p. 65

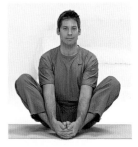

Butterfly, p. 68

main exercises

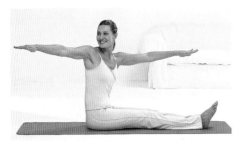

Pilates Spinal Twist, p. 83

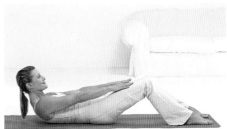

Roll Up, p. 90–91

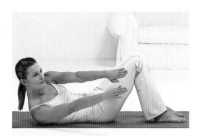

Diagonal Curl Up, p. 92

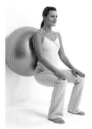

Wall Squat, p. 105

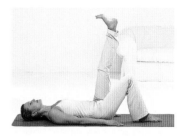

Single-Leg Raise, p. 86

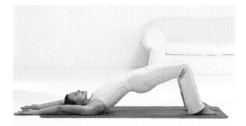

The Bridge (variation), p. 96

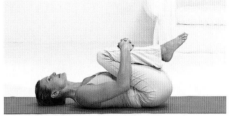

Double-Leg Stretch, p. 97

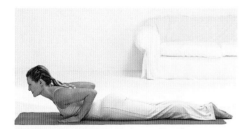

Swan Dive, p. 98–99

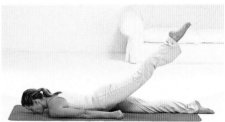

Prone Leg Raise, p 101

cool down

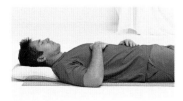

Progressive Relaxation, p. 76–77, or
Rhythmic Diaphragmatic Breathing, p. 78

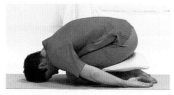

or in Child's Pose, p. 79

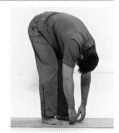

or Roll Down, p. 74–75

shortened programmes – advanced

warm-ups

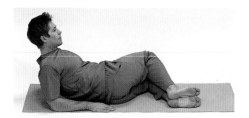

Lying Twist (variation), p. 70

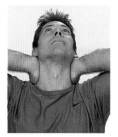

Neck Stretch, p. 65

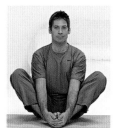

Butterfly, p. 68

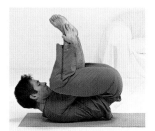

Seal, p. 73

main exercises

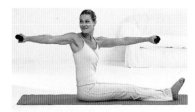

Pilates Spinal Twist (advanced), p. 83

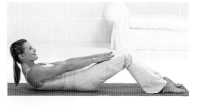

Roll Up, p. 90–91

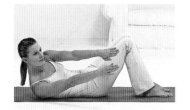

Diagonal Curl Up (with or without ball), p. 92

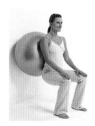

Wall Squat, p. 105

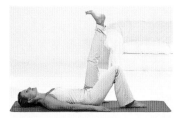

Single-Leg Raise, p. 86

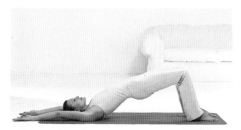

The Bridge (variation), p. 96

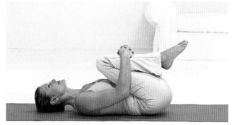

Double-Leg Stretch, p. 97

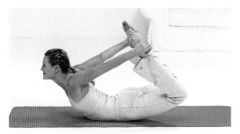

Rocking, p. 100

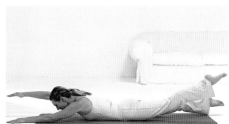

Swimming, p. 101

cool down

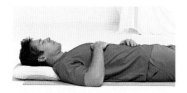

Progressive Relaxation, p. 76–77, or
Rhythmic Diaphragmatic Breathing, p. 78

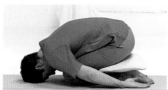

or in Child's Pose, p. 79

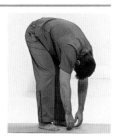

or Roll Down, p. 74–75

pregnancy

NOTE

Please consult the list of cautions on pages 62–63 before attempting this exercise programme.

warm-ups

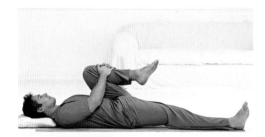

Single-Knee Hug, p. 69

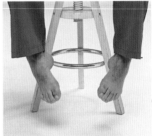

Foot Circles, p. 67

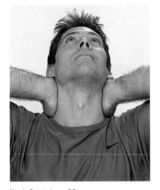

Neck Stretch, p. 65

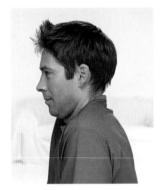

Shoulder Circle p. 66

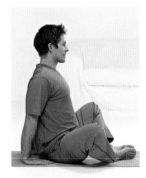

Butterfly (variation), p. 68

main exercises

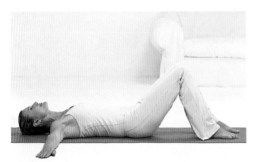

Pelvic Tilt, p. 93

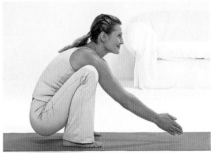

Squatting, p. 105

main exercises continued

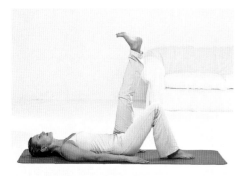

Single-Leg Raise, p. 86

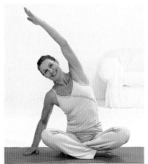

Sideways Stretch, p. 82

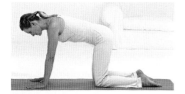

Cat Stretch, p. 104

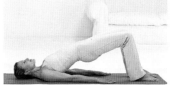

The Bridge, p. 96

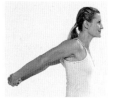

Chest Expansion,p. 80

cool down

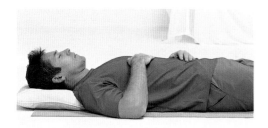

Progressive Relaxation, p. 76–77, or Rhythmic
Diaphragmatic Breathing, p. 78

glossary

Anterior Before or in front of

Cervical Pertaining to the region of the neck

Coccyx Small bone at the base of the spinal column (also known as the 'tailbone')

Diaphragm Muscular dome-shaped partition separating the chest and abdominal cavities

Endorphins Chemicals produced in the brain involved in pain perception; the body's natural pain relievers

Extend Movement that brings a limb into or towards a straight condition; opposite of flex

Facets Bony surfaces of the rear part of a vertebra that match up with similar surfaces on neighbouring vertebrae and guide their movements

Flex Bend upon itself. Bend a joint or limb; the opposite of extend

Hamstrings Three muscles on the back of the thigh (also known as the semitendinosus).

Intervertebral disc Broad, flattened disc of fibrocartilage between the bodies of vertebrae

Kyphosis Refers to a spinal curve that is convex towards the rear

Ligament A band of fibrous tissue connecting bones forming a joint

Lordosis Refers to a spinal curve that is convex towards the front

Lumbar Pertaining to the loins; the part of the back between the chest and the pelvis

Osteoporosis A disease characterized by low bone mass and structural deterioration of the bone tissue

Pelvic floor A muscular sling-like support for the pelvic organs; situated at the bottom of the pelvis

Perineum The tissues between the anus and the genitals

Pilates stance The V position of the feet, heels together and toes a few inches apart. See also Tripod position

Posterior Placed at the back

Prone Lying horizontal with the face downwards; the opposite of supine

Sacroiliac joints The joints formed by the hip bones and the sacrum

Sacrum A triangular bone located at the back of the pelvis; made up of five fused vertebrae

Semitendinosus Hamstring muscles

Spondylolisthesis A forward slipping of the lower lumbar vertebrae on the sacrum

Spondylolysis A separation or break in the vertebral bone

Supine Lying on the back with the face upwards; the opposite of prone

Tendon A band of fibrous tissue forming the end of a muscle and attaching it to a bone

Thoracic Pertaining to the chest

Torsion Twisting

Tripod position A Pilates stance in which body weight is distributed equally over three points: the ball of the foot, the middle of the heel and the outside edge of the foot, near the little toe

Vertebra Any one of the 33 bones (vertebrae) forming the spinal column

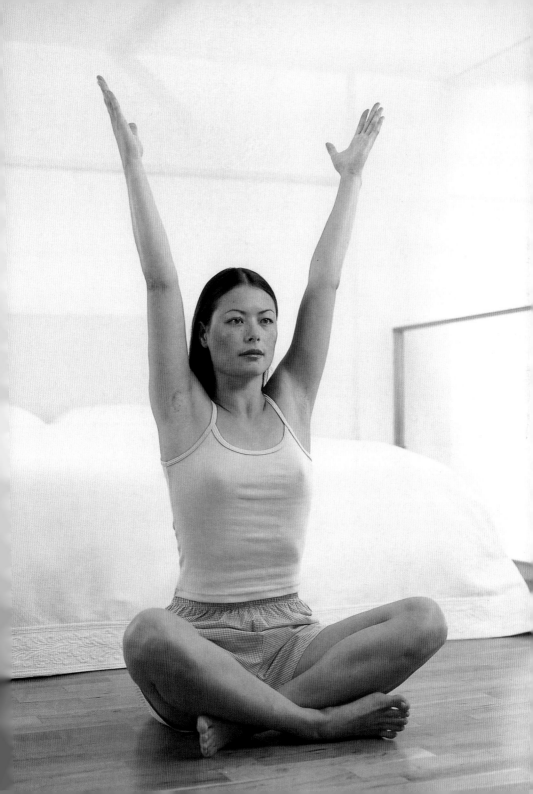

index

A

abdominal muscles 15, 24
  diagonal curl up 92
  little abdominal curl 88–9
  roll up 90–1
  teaser 94–5
acupressure 34–5
acupuncture 34–5
adductor muscle 15
advanced programme 112–13,
  118–19
ageing 18, 24
air travel 49
Alexander Technique 35, 55
anaesthetics, local 31
analgesics 30
anatomy 10–17
ankylosing spondylitis 20
anorexia nervosa 23
anti-anxiety breath 39
antidepressants 30–1
anxiety 39
arm circle with weights 67
arthritis 20
articular processes, vertebrae 12
aspirin 30, 31

B

back, lying on 40, 41
back pain 6
  breathing 38–9
  causes of 18–25
  chronic pain 24, 43
  managing 27–43
  pain control 28–9
  and pelvic floor 17
  prevention 45–57
  relaxation 36–7
  responses to 23–4, 28

rest positions 40–1
risk factors 24–5
self-help 29, 42–3
treatment 30–5
backbone see spine
balls, Swiss 56–7, 61
  lying twist with ball 71
  wall squat 105
bed rest 40, 41
beginners programme 108–9,
  114–15
biofeedback, pain control 29, 36–7
body mechanics 46–7
bones
  osteoporosis 22, 54
  pelvic ring 16
  spine 10
brain 11
breathing
  pain control 38–9
  rhythmic diaphragmatic
    breathing 78–9
the bridge 96
butterfly 68

C

carrying heavy loads 50
cars, driving 47
cartilage, intervertebral discs 13
cat stretch 104
cervical vertebrae 10, 13
chest expansion 80
'chi', acupuncture 34
child's pose 79
chin glide 64
Chinese medicine 34–5
chiropractic 35
chronic pain 24
  treatment 43

clothing 61
coccyx 10
cold treatment 28, 31–2
complementary therapies 29
compression, vertebrae 24
cooling down 74–9
  advanced programme 113, 119
  beginners programme 108, 115
  intermediate programme 111,
    117
  in pregnancy 121
corticosteroid injections 31
curls
  diagonal curl up 92
  little abdominal curl 88–9
curves, spine 11, 16, 20
  kyphosis 20, 22
  scoliosis 22
cyclobenzaprine 30

D

daily activities, posture 50–1
degenerative changes 18
depression 30–1
diagonal curl up 92
diaphragmatic breathing 38, 78–9
diet 43
discs
  discectomy 31
  intervertebral 13, 18–19
distraction, pain control 29
divided breath 39
dog stretch 102
double-leg stretch 97
driving, posture 47
drugs 30–1, 42

E

electrical therapy 33

emergencies 43
endorphins 28, 33, 54
energy, acupuncture, 34-5
equipment 61
erector spinae muscle 15
exercise
    guidelines 60–1
    preventing back pain 54
    safety 61, 62–3
exercise balls 56–7, 61
    lying twist with ball 71
    wall squat 105
external oblique muscles 15

F
facet joints 12, 21
    compression of vertebrae 24
feet
    foot circles 67
    reflexology 29
Feldenkrais Method 29
femur 16
Flexeril 30
foot circles 67
foramina 11
fractures, osteoporosis 22, 54

G
gastrocnemius muscle 15
'gate control' theory, pain control
    28–9, 33
getting up, safety 41
gluteus maximus muscle 15
golf 48

H
half moon 82
hamstrings 15
healing visualization 37
heat treatment 28, 32
herniated discs 18–19
hip bones 10, 16

hip joints 16
hormones, in pregnancy 23
hunchback (kyphosis) 20, 22

I
ibuprofen 30, 31
ice treatment 31–2
ilium 10
illness, exercise after 75
imagery, pain control 37
inactivity, and back pain 23
infections 22
inflammation 30, 31
injections, corticosteroid 31
injuries 20–1, 25
innominate bones 16
intermediate programme 110–11,
    116–17
internal oblique muscles 15
intervertebral discs 13
    back pain 18–19
    compression of vertebrae 24
    surgery 31
intervertebral joints 12

J
Jacobson, Edmund 40
joints
    arthritis 20
    and back pain 23
    benefits of exercise 54
    chiropractic 35
    intervertebral 12
    osteopathy 35
    pelvic ring 16
    in pregnancy 23

K
kyphosis (hunchback) 20, 22

L
laminectomy 31

latissimus dorsi muscle 15
Leboyer, Dr Frederick 23–4
legs
    muscles 15
    prone leg raise 101
    sciatica 18
    single-leg kicks 103
    single-leg raise 86–7
lifting safety 52–3
ligaments 14
    and back pain 23
    injuries 21
    pelvic floor 17
    pelvic ring 16
    in pregnancy 23
    traction 28
little abdominal curl 88–9
lumbar spine, injuries 21
lumbar vertebrae 10, 12
    compression of 24
    spondylolisthesis 21
lying down, rest positions 40–1
lying twist 70
lying twist with ball 71

M
manipulation 35
massage 28, 33
medicines 30–1, 42
Melzack, Ronald 28, 33
meridians, acupuncture, 34
muscles
    abdominal muscles 15, 24
    and back pain 23
    benefits of exercise 54
    and chronic pain 24
    cooling down 74–9
    injuries 20–1
    leg muscles 15
    pelvic floor muscles 17
    Progressive Relaxation 40,
        76–7

relaxant drugs 30
rest 42
spinal support muscles 14, 15
traction 28
warming up 60, 64–73

N

neck
chin glide 64
neck stretch 65
vertebrae 10
nerves 11
back pain 21
chiropractic 35
'gate control' theory 28–9, 33
TENS machines 33
NSAIDs (non-steroidal anti-
inflammatory drugs) 30

O

occupations
and back pain 25
posture 47
osteoarthritis 20
osteopathy 35
osteoporosis 22, 54
overweight, and back pain 23

P

pain see back pain
Palmer, Daniel David 35
paracetamol 30
pelvis
abdominal muscles 15
pelvic floor muscles 17
pelvic ring 16
pelvic tilt 93
perineal exercise 17
perineum 17
perineal exercise 17
physical therapy, back pain 28
physiotherapy 43

Pilates 56
Pilates spine twist 83
posture 15, 16
Alexander Technique 35, 55
body mechanics 46–7
checking 46
and chronic back pain 24
daily activities 50–1
herniated discs and 18
sports 48–9
posture clasp 81
pregnancy
effects on back 23, 25
exercising during 62–3, 120–1
preventing back pain 45–57
processes, vertebrae 12
Progressive Relaxation 40, 76–7
prolapsed discs 18–19
prone leg raise 101
prostaglandins 31
psychological pain control 29
'pulled muscles' 20
pulling and pushing, safety 50

Q

quadriceps muscle 15
quadriceps stretch 103

R

rectus abdominis muscle 15
reflexology 29
relaxation
biofeedback 36
pain control 29
Progressive Relaxation 40,
76–7
rest positions 40–1
self-help for pain 43
visualization and imagery 37
relaxin 23
rest 40–1, 42
rheumatoid arthritis 20

rhythmic diaphragmatic
breathing 78–9
ribs, abdominal muscles 15
risk factors, back pain 24–5
rocking 100
Rolfing 29
roll down 74–5
roll up 90–1
rolling
rolling like a ball 72
seal 73

S

sacral vertebrae 10
sacroiliac joint 10
injuries 21
pelvic ring 16
in pregnancy 23
sacrum 10, 13
pelvic ring 16
spondylolisthesis 21
safety 61, 62–3
sciatica 18
scoliosis 22
seal 73
self-help, pain control 29, 42–3
semitendinosus muscle 15
sexual positions 51
shoes, and chronic back pain 24,
43
shortened programmes 114–19
shoulders
chest expansion, 80
posture clasp 81
shoulder circle 66
sideways stretch 82
single-knee hug 69
single-leg kicks 103
single-leg raise 86–7
sitting
and back pain 23
and chronic back pain 24

posture 46
skiing 49
sleep problems 54
slipped discs 13, 18
spasm, muscular 20–1
spinal canal 12
spinal cord 10, 11, 21
spinal fusion 31
spine
    anatomy 10–17
    back pain 18–25
    curves 11, 16, 20
    intervertebral discs 13, 18–19
    ligaments 14
    muscles 14, 15
    pelvic ring 16
    tendons 14
    vertebrae 10, 12
spondylolisthesis 21–2
spondylolysis 22
spondylosis 20
sports
    injuries 18, 20, 25
    posture 48–9
sprains 21
squatting 105
    wall squat 105
Still, Andrew Taylor 35
strains 20–1
stress, and back pain 23–4
stretches
    cat stretch 104
    dog stretch 102
    double-leg stretch 97
    neck stretch 65
    quadriceps stretch 103
    sideways stretch 82
    warming up 21
suggestion, pain control 29
surgery 18, 31
swan dive 98–9
swimming exercise 101

Swiss balls 56–7, 61
    lying twist with ball 71
    wall squat 105
symphysis pubis 16
symptoms questionnaire 25

T
tailbone 10
tears, muscles 20–1
teaser 94–5
tendons 14
tennis 49
TENS (transcutaneous electric
    nerve stimulation) 33
thigh bone 16
thoracic spine, kyphosis 20
thoracic vertebrae 10
traction 28
transverse processes, vertebrae
    12
transversus abdominis muscle 15
trapezius muscle 15
travel, posture 49
tumours 22
turtle 64
twists
    lying twist 70
    lying twist with ball 71
    Pilates spine twist 83
    safety 51
    yoga spinal twist 84–5

U
ultrasound treatment 33–4

V
vertebrae 10, 12
    compression of 24
    facet joints 12, 21
    intervertebral discs 13, 18–19
    ligaments 14
    osteoporosis 22

spondylolisthesis 21–2
spondylolysis 22
surgery 31
vertebral column see spine
visualization
    pain control 37, 61
    perineal exercise 17

W
Wall, Patrick 28, 33
wall squat 105
warming up 21, 43, 60, 64–73
    advanced programme 112, 118
    beginners programme 108, 114
    intermediate programme 110,
    116
    in pregnancy 120
weight, and back pain 23
weights 61
    arm circle with weights 67
work
    and back pain 25
    posture 47

Y
yoga 38–9, 40, 57
yoga spinal twist 84–5

acknowledgements

Many thanks to everyone who has contributed to this book. I am particularly grateful to Jane McIntosh, Jessica Cowie, Harriet Stewart-Jones and Nikki Sims. Special thanks go to David for so generously sharing his computer expertise; to Walter for his unwavering support and many hours at the computer, and to Karl for his contribution to chapter 1 and, along with Lora, for his continued interest and encouragement.

Executive Editor Jane McIntosh
Managing Editor Clare Churly
Executive Art Editor Mark Stevens
Designer Ginny Zeal
Production Manager Ian Paton
Picture Research Sophie Delpech
Illustrator Trevor Bounford

picture acknowledgements

All photography: © Octopus Publishing Group Limited/Mike Prior, with the following exceptions: **Alamy**/Imageshop/Benno de Wilde 23. **Digital Vision** 20. **Getty Images**/James Darell 7, 24. **Octopus Publishing Group Limited** 30; /Alistair Hughes 51; /Angus Murray 48; /Peter Pugh-Cook 38, 42, 54, 55, 56, 57 top left, 62, 63, 76; /Russell Sadur 57 bottom right, 123; /Ian Wallace 32, 34; /Mark Winwood 36. **Photodisc** 21. **Shutterstock**/Olga Utlyakova 49.